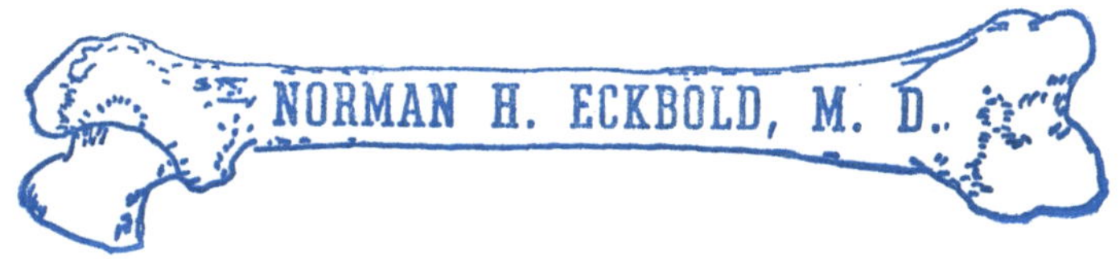

NORMAN H. ECKBOLD, M. D.

AF251027

MRI of the Shoulder

MRI of the Shoulder

Clinical Situations and Management

Michael Shannon
Pietro Tonino

145 illustrations

1992
Georg Thieme Verlag Stuttgart · New York
Thieme Medical Publishers, Inc. New York

Michael Shannon, M. D.
Assistant Professor of Radiology
Loyola University of Chicago
and
Associate Radiologist
Berwyn Magnetic Resonance Center
3345 S. Oak Park Ave.
Berwyn, IL 60402
USA

Pietro Tonino, M. D.
Assistant Professor of Orthopedic Surgery
Chief, Section of Sports Medicine
Loyola University Medical Center
2160 S. First Ave.
Maywood, IL 60153
USA

Library of Congress Cataloging-in-Publication Data

Shannon, Michael.
MRI of the shoulder : clinical situations and management / Michael Shannon, Pietro Tonino.
    p.   cm.
Includes bibliographical references and index.
1. Shoulder—Magnetic resonance imaging. I. Tonino, Pietro.
II. Title.
[DNLM: 1. Joint Diseases—diagnosis. 2. Magnetic Resonance Imaging. 3. Shoulder Joint. WE 810 S528m]
RC939.S47   1991
617.5'7207548—dc20
DNLM/DLC

Important Note: Medicine is an ever-changing science undergoing continual development. Research and clinical experience are continually expanding our knowledge, in particular our knowledge of proper treatment and drug therapy. Insofar as this book mentions any dosage or application, readers may rest assured that the authors, editors and publishers have made every effort to ensure that such references are in accordance with the state of knowledge at the time of production of the book.
Nevertheless this does not involve, imply, or express any guarantee or responsibility on the part of the publishers in respect of any dosage instructions and forms of application stated in the book. Every user is requested to examine carefully the manufacturers' leaflets accompanying each drug and to check, if necessary in consultation with a physician or specialist, whether the dosage schedules mentioned therein or the contraindications stated by the manufacturers differ from the statements made in the present book. Such examination is particularly important with drugs that are either rarely used or have been newly released on the market. Every dosage schedule or every form of application used is entirely at the user's own risk and responsibility. The authors and publishers request every user to report to the publishers any discrepancies or inaccuracies noticed.

© 1992 Georg Thieme Verlag,
Rüdigerstraße 14, D-7000 Stuttgart 30
Thieme Medical Publishers, Inc., 381 Park Avenue South, New York, N. Y. 10016

Typesetting by Karl Lihs, D-7140 Ludwigsburg
(Linotype System 4/300)

Printed in Germany by Karl Grammlich,
D-7401 Pliezhausen

ISBN 3-13-774001-0 (GTV, Stuttgart)
ISBN 0-86577-419-6 (TMP, New York)

1   2   3   4   5   6

Preface

The past 10 to 15 years have seen an increased emphasis on physical activity and competitive sports in all segments of the population. This is, of course, a favorable trend, but the downside of it is an increase in joint and musculoskeletal problems. Because of the popularity of jogging and aerobics, and because running is a feature of most competitive and team sports, the knee is the most-afflicted joint. The shoulder is arguably the second most frequently impaired joint in sports activity. Physical laborers required to do heavy lifting and construction workers also have a high incidence of shoulder complaints. In the rising population of the elderly, injuries to the tendons around the shoulder joint are common, even with ordinary activities.

It is fortunate that magnetic resonance imaging (MRI) has become available at a time in which shoulder pathology is more frequently seen. It is a noninvasive procedure that does not use ionizing radiation. It provides detailed visualization of soft-tissue structures that is not possible with other imaging modalities. Though not as widely available as conventional radiographs or computed tomography (CT) scanning, the number of MRI units worldwide is increasing steadily. The development of surface coils specifically for the shoulder has greatly improved the quality of the images in the last several years.

Imaging techniques should not be a substitue for a thorough patient history and physical examination. Determination of which patients will have pathologic changes of the shoulder likely to be demonstrated in MRI is important in this era of increasing medical expenditures and cost containment.

This monograph does not attempt to be a comprehensive study of shoulder pathology. It presents a variety of conditions commonly seen with shoulder injury and their appearance on MRI.

Michael Shannon, M. D.
Pietro Tonino, M. D.

Acknowledgments

The help and encouragement of Dr. Galdino Valvassori in preparing this book is greatly appreciated. Support has been provided by Dr. Glen Dobben and Medical Systems of the General Electric Company, Milwaukee, Wisconsin. The technologists and staff of the Berwyn Magnetic Resonance Center, Berwyn, Illinois, have aided in the completion of this project.

Further assistance has also been provided by Patricia Flanagan, Department of Orthopedics, Loyola University Medical Center, Maywood, Illinois.

Contents

1 The Physical Basis of Magnetic Resonance Imaging

Magnetic resonance imaging (MRI) takes advantage of the behavior of the protons in the nuclei of atoms with an odd atomic number in the presence of high magnetic fields. The hydrogen atom is the most abundant element in organic tissue and at this time is almost exclusively used in all MRI.

The hydrogen nucleus, made up of a single proton, behaves like a small spinning magnet. The directions of the spins of the nuclei are randomly oriented under normal circumstances, but in the presence of a superimposed magnetic field they become oriented in a direction parallel or antiparallel to the magnetic field (Fig. 1.**1**). The parallel orientation is a relatively lower energy state than the antiparallel direction. The nuclei spin about an axis aligned to the magnetic field. The rate at which the nuclei spin about the axis is proportional to the strength of the magnetic field.

If a second magnetic field is suddenly applied to the system, the axes of the spins of the hydrogen nuclei will become reoriented with their spins about an axis parallel to this new field. Energy is required by the nuclei to change their spin direction and this energy is derived from the new magnetic field. For the energy to be absorbed by the hydrogen nuclei, the frequency of rotation of the magnetic field must be the same as the spin rate of the hydrogen nuclei (the Larmour frequency). The frequency of rotation of the hydrogen protons is of a magnitude similar to the frequency of radio waves in the electromagnetic spectrum. For this reason, the transverse magnetic field is sometimes referred to as the RF. The length of time the new field is applied to the system will determine the angle of displacement of the nuclei from their orientation to the original magnetic field. The nuclei can be reoriented to an axis at a 90° or 180° angle to the original direction, or at any other angle (Fig. 1.**2**).

When the transverse magnetic field is discontinued, the hydrogen nuclei revert to the

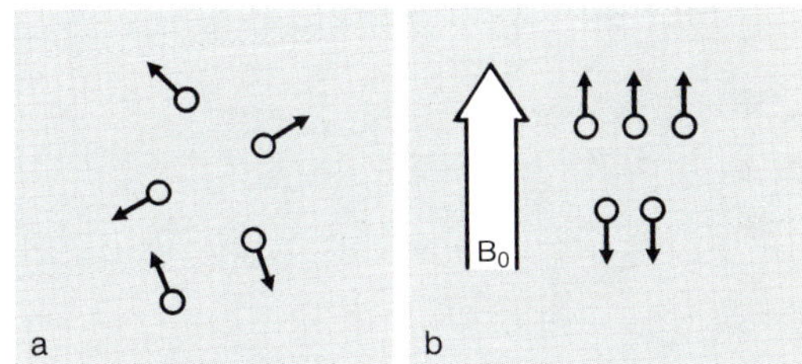

Fig. 1.**1a** Hydrogen protons are depicted by circles and the spin direction of each by an arrow. Normally the protons spin in random directions

Fig. 1.**1b** In the presence of a superimposed magnetic field (B_0), the spins of the protons will become oriented in a direction parallel, or slightly less frequently, anti-parallel, to the direction of the magnetic field. The protons spin at a characteristic rate that is proportional to the strength of the magnetic field

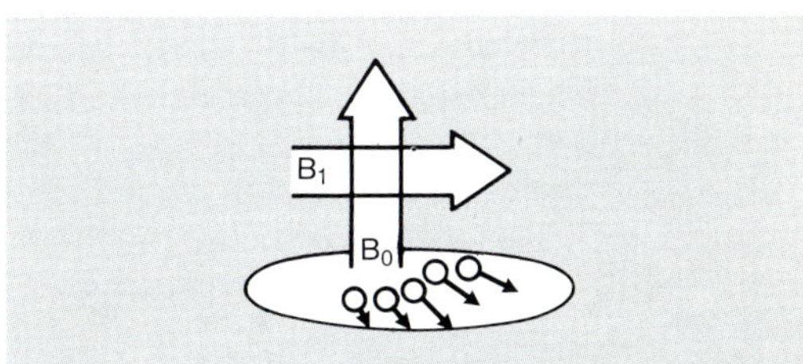

Fig. 1.**2** A second magnetic field (B_1) is superimposed in a direction perpendicular to B_0, rotating at a frequency which matches the rate of spins of the protons long enough to flip the spin directions of the protons 90°

orientation of the originally applied magnetic field, returning to the original, lower energy state. Energy is released in the process of reorientation, and this energy can induce an electric current in a receiving coil which is proportional in strength to the energy dissipated. This is the principle of the signal which is received in MRI and allows the production of the images.

In reverting to the energy state that existed before superimposition of the transverse

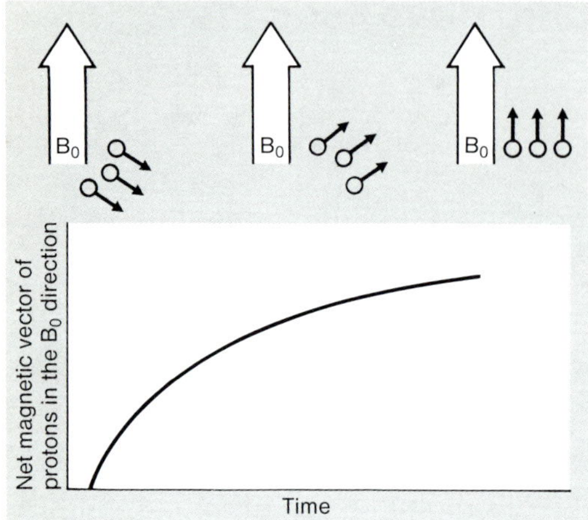

Fig. 1.3   When magnetic field B_1 is discontinued, the magnetic vector of the protons in the direction of B_0 is zero. Over time, the net magnetic vector in the B_0 direction increases exponentially as the protons regain that orientation. This is T1 relaxation

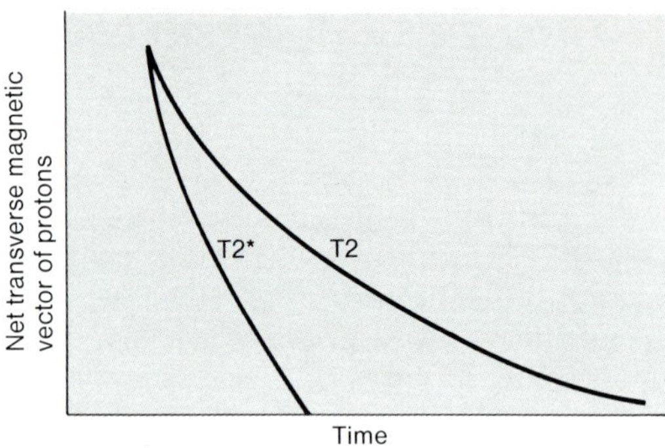

Fig. 1.4a   T2 relaxation is a measure of the dissipation of the magnetic vector of the protons in the transverse (B_1) direction caused by the development of asynchronism in the spins of the protons. The net magnetic vector in this direction should decrease exponentially to zero at time T2. In reality, the net magnetic vector decreases much faster, in a time T2*, because of local inhomogeneities in the magnetic field

magnetic field, the hydrogen nuclei undergo two forms of dissipation of the excess energy, or relaxation. At the termination of the RF, the affected hydrogen nuclei will have zero magnetic orientation in the direction of the original field. Over a given time, usually measured in milliseconds, the net magnetic vector will exponentially increase in the direction of the original field as the protons realign parallel to the original field (Fig. 1.3). This is called T1 relaxation.

Depletion of the induced transverse magnetic field of the protons also occurs as their spins become out of phase with one another when the RF pulse is discontinued. Ideally, the synchronism of the spins and the transverse magnetic vector of the protons would decline exponentially. This is called T2 relaxation. In reality, however, the synchronism declines much more rapidly because the individual protons are influenced by small differences in their local magnetic fields. The time measured for this actual decrease in the transverse synchronism of spins is called T2* and is shorter than T2 (Fig. 1.4a). In order to reduce the effects of these local magnetic inhomogeneities, which degrade the signal received, a second transverse magnetic field is applied some time after the first. This second pulse is turned on

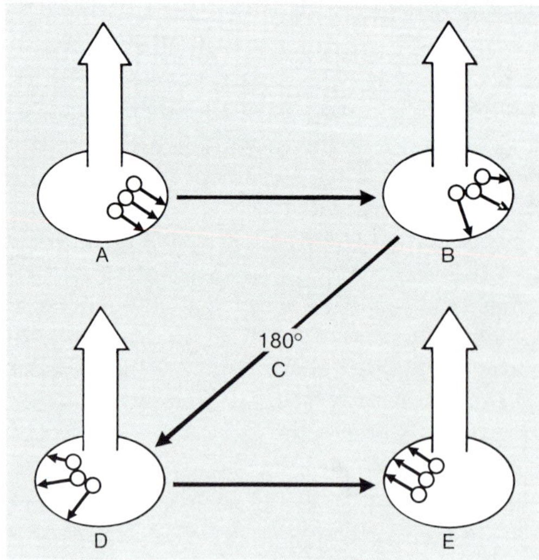

Fig. 1.4b   (A) The protons spin in phase immediately after the RF pulse. (B) Their spins gradually become dephased, the faster spins displayed by longer arrows. (C) A second RF pulse long enough to produce a 180° flip of the protons in the transverse plane is applied. (D) The protons are still out of phase, but those with the faster spins are now positioned behind the slower. (E) At a time interval that is twice the interval between the 90° and 180° pulses, the spins again are briefly in phase, and the signal is obtained

long enough to produce a 180° change of direction of the transverse magnetization. This has the effect of refocusing the asynchronous spins of the protons (Fig. 1.**4b**). A stronger signal can then be obtained with fewer artifacts in the images. This is called a spin-echo imaging sequence, and is widely used in MRI of all parts of the body. The time between the 90° pulse and the readout (reception of the signal) is twice the amount of time between the 90° and 180° pulses and is called the echo time (TE). The time between a 90° pulse and application of the next 90° pulse for the next image of a sequence is called the repetition time (TR; Fig. 1.**5**).

The T1, as we have seen, is a measure of the dissipation of the transverse magnetization after the 90° RF pulse. A tissue that has an intrinsically short T1 will demonstrate a more rapid return of the magnetic vector aligned to the direction of the original magnetic field than a tissue with a longer T1. Therefore, when the next 90° pulse is applied, it will affect a larger number of protons (Fig. 1.**6**). This will only be true if the TR is relatively short in relation to the T1 relaxation times of the tissues involved, because as the TR becomes longer, more of the protons of both the long and short T1 tissues will have returned to the original magnetic vector (Fig. 1.**7**). Therefore, the TR determines the degree of T1 dependence of an image. Since the TE cannot be longer than the TR in an imaging sequence, a short TE and a short TR will produce a T1-weighted image. The tissues with the shorter T1 relaxation times will have the stronger (brighter) signal on a T1-weighted image.

T2 is a measure of the speed with which asynchronism develops in the spins of the 90°-tipped protons. If a tissue has a long intrinsic T2 value, the protons will be only slightly out of phase when the refocusing 180° pulse arrives, and will have a strong signal. With a short T2, the spins will become more asynchronous before the 180° pulse, and will not refocus as readily, thus giving a weaker signal (Fig. 1.**8**). The TE will determine the relative T2 weighting of a sequence. If the TE is too short, transverse magnetization will be similar in tissue with long or short T2's. With a longer TE, the various tissues will have degrees of

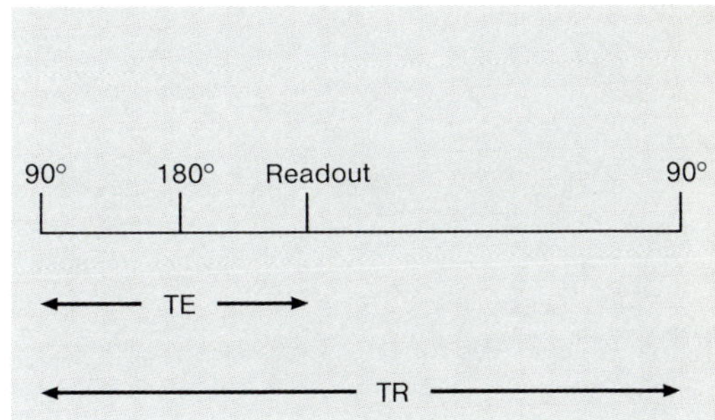

Fig. 1.**5** The time between the 90° RF pulse and the readout is called the echo time (TE). The time between a 90° pulse and the next 90° pulse for the image is called the repetition time (TR)

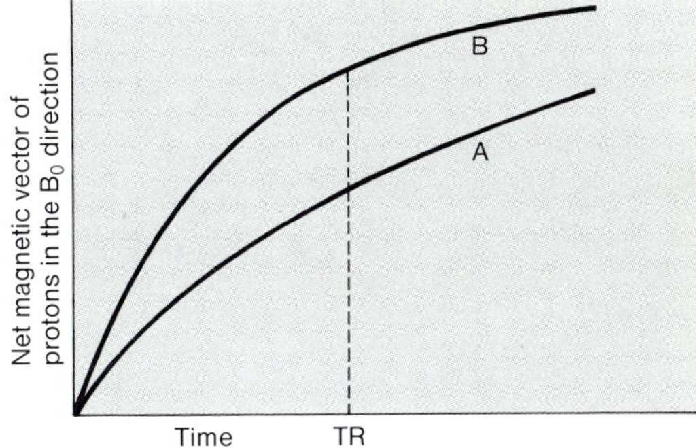

Fig. 1.**6** The graph depicts the T1 relaxation of two different tissues, A and B. Tissue B has a shorter T1 than tissue A. At time TR, more protons from tissue B will have returned to their original magnetic orientation, and will be available to be excited by the next 90° pulse, producing a stronger signal. A tissue with a short T1 has a higher signal than one with a long T1

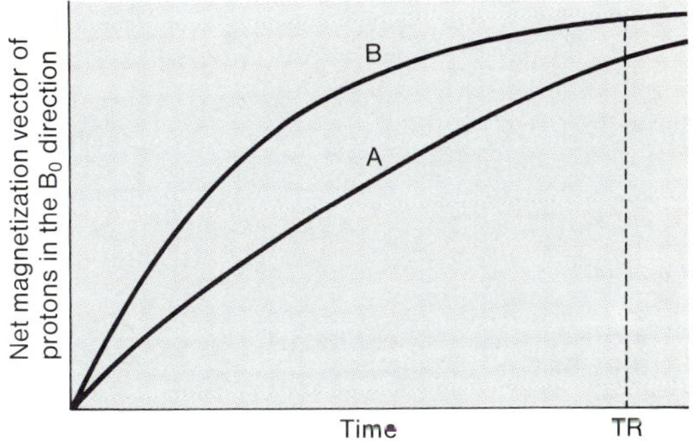

Fig. 1.**7** The T1 relaxation of two different tissues is shown on the graph. Tissue B has a shorter T1 than tissue A. If the TR is very long in relation to the T1 values, however, both tissues will have resumed their original states by the time the next 90° pulse arrives, and T1 will have little influence on the strength of the signal

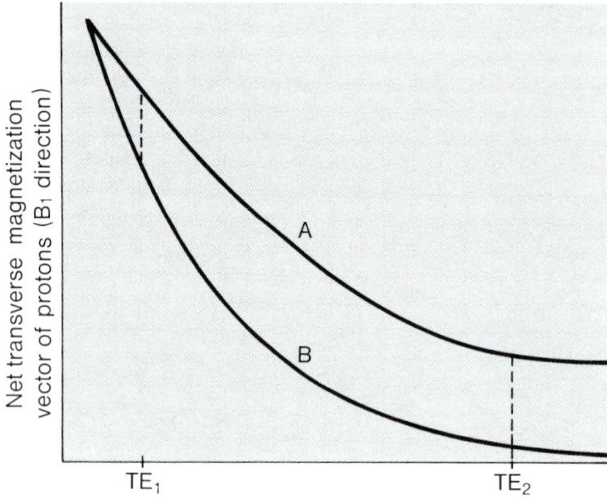

Fig. 1.8 The graph depicts the T2 relaxation of tissue A (slower), and tissue B (faster). If the TE is short relative to T2 (as at time TE_1), there will be little signal difference between the two tissues. If the TE is longer (as at time TE_2), signal difference between the two tissues will be increased

Table 1.1 Signal intensity received as dependent on the intrinsic T1 and T2 values

	Short	Long
T1	Bright	Dark
T2	Dark	Bright

Table 1.2 Relative time intervals for TE and TR for T1, proton-density, and T2 images

	TE	TR
T1	Short	Short
Proton density	Short	Long
T2	Long	Long

Table 1.3 Signal intensities of various types of tissue on T1- and T2-weighted images

	T1	T2
Fat	Bright	Less bright
Fluid (serous)	Low intermediate	Bright
Muscle	Intermediate (gray)	Intermediate
Fibrous tissue	Dark	Dark
Bone (cortex)	Dark	Dark

difference in their residual transverse magnetic strengths, and the effect on the images will be maximized (Fig. 1.8). Therefore, a long TE will cause T2 weighting of the images. The TR cannot be shorter than the TE, so a long TE

and a long TR produce strongly T2-weighted images. A tissue with a long T2 will have a stronger (brighter) signal than one with a short T2. (Tables 1.1, 1.2).

If a short TE is used in a sequence with a long TR, all tissue will return to the original magnetization state between successive 90° pulses. The signal differences between various tissues will then be influenced by the number of protons affected. Denser tissues will exhibit a stronger signal than less compact tissues because more protons per unit volume will be available for excitation and signal production. This type of sequence produces proton density–weighted images. A proton-density sequence is frequently performed with a T2 sequence by inducing a 180° pulse first with a short TE, and then a second 180° pulse with a longer TE between each successive TR.

Each type of body tissue has its own value of T1 and T2 relaxation times depending on the state of molecular bonding of the hydrogen atoms. The differences thus allow the discrimination of the various tissues in MRI. Tissue distinction is much more precise than on conventional radiographs and computed tomography (CT) scans. Table 1.3 lists the signal intensities of various tissues on images obtained with T1 and T2 weighting.

Cortical bone has a low signal intensity because the hydrogen atoms are tightly bound, and not free to change their spin orientation, thus giving no signal. Fat has a high signal on T1-weighted images because the protons quickly revert to the original magnetic field orientation after the 90° pulse is removed (a short T1). Serous fluid, like a simple joint effusion, has a high signal on T2-weighted images because the spins of the protons only slowly become asynchronous after the 90° pulse is removed (a long T2).

References

Curry TS, Dowdey JE, Murry RC. Christensen's physics of diagnostic radiology. 4th ed. Philadelphia: Lea & Febiger, 1990: 432–504.

Kean DM, Smith MA. Magnetic resonance imaging: principles and applications. Baltimore: Williams & Wilkins, 1986: 6–69.

Stark DD, Bradley WG. Magnetic resonance imaging. St. Louis: C.V. Mosby, 1988: 3–55.

2 Normal Shoulder Anatomy and MR Imaging

The shoulder joint is comprised of the head of the humerus articulating with the glenoid fossa of the scapula. The glenoid fossa is a shallow smooth concave surface with a much larger potential radius of its curvature than the much smaller radius of the humeral head. This lack of conformity of their surfaces allows for the joint to have a great range of motion. The curvature of the glenoid fossa is deepened slightly by a rim of fibrocartilage, the glenoidal labrum, which is attached around its circumference.

The wide range of motion of the shoulder joint is further allowed by the looseness of the joint capsule. The capsule is a thin fibrous structure covering the synovial lining of the joint. Medially it attaches around the circumference of the glenoid and laterally to the neck and shaft of the humerus. The capsule is strengthened by three, or variably two, glenohumeral ligaments which are thick bands on its anterior aspect. Inferiorly, the joint space forms a loose pouch, the axillary recess. The redundancy of the axillary recess allows the extreme positions of shoulder motion. The joint capsule becomes more taut when the arm is held at 180° of elevation.

There are five intrinsic muscles of the shoulder joint, which are muscles extending only from the scapula to the humerus. Four of these, the supraspinatus, the infraspinatus, the subscapularis, and the teres minor, make up the musculotendinous cuff, more commonly called the rotator cuff. The fifth intrinsic muscle is the teres major, which is not part of the rotator cuff (Fig. 2.**1**).

The supraspinatus forms the upper portion of the rotator cuff. Its origin is on the flat supraspinatus fossa on the posterior side of the scapula, above the scapular spine. It extends laterally and anteriorly across the upper joint capsule. The muscular fibers gradually coalesce with the flat tendon of the muscle on the upper aspect of the humeral head. The tendon inserts onto the upper facet of the greater tuberosity (Fig. 2.**1b**). The tendon of the supraspinatus blends with the fibrous outer aspect of the joint capsule and reinforces it. The merging muscle and tendon fibers pass beneath the acromion process. A subacromial

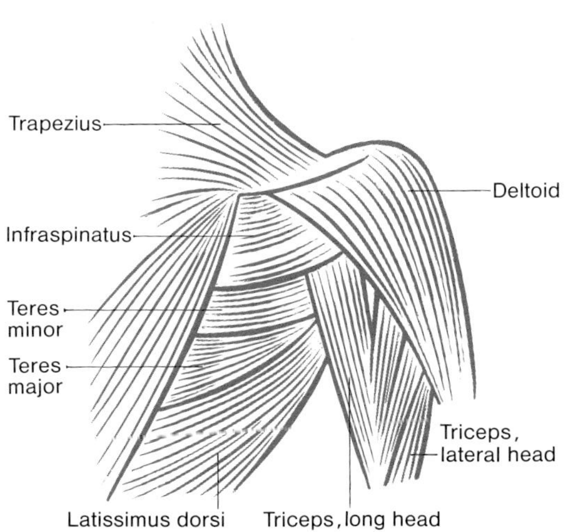

Fig. 2.**1 a** Posterior view of the superficial muscles of the shoulder

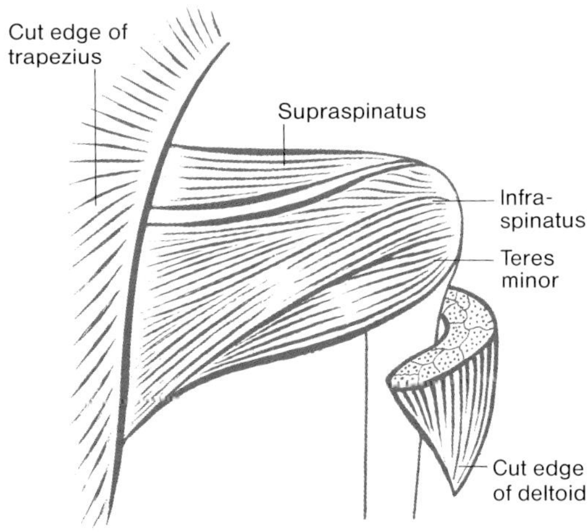

Fig. 2.**1 b** Posterior view of the deep muscles of the shoulder

bursa, which does not normally communicate with the shoulder joint, lies between the tendon and the acromion.

The infraspinatus originates on the medial two-thirds of the infraspinatus fossa of the scapula. Its tendon extends around the posterior side of the humeral head to insert on the greater tuberosity just below the supraspinatus (Fig. 2.**1b**). A bursa may be present between the tendon and the humerus, and this bursa usually does communicate with the joint space.

The teres minor arises from the upper two-thirds of the axillary margin of the scapula below the scapular spine. This muscle parallels the infraspinatus, and inserts just below the latter on the greater tuberosity of the humerus (Fig. 2.**1b**). It may not be distinguishable from the infraspinatus on MR images.

The fourth intrinsic shoulder muscle, and the last of the rotator cuff muscles, is the subscapularis. It originates on the front of the scapula, from the subscapular fossa. Its tendon extends anterolaterally across the anterior aspect of the humeral head. It is the only muscle of the rotator cuff to insert on the lesser tuberosity of the humerus (Fig. 2.**2**). A bursa deep to this muscle usually communicates with the joint space.

The tendon of the long head of the biceps originates from a protuberance on the superior rim of the glenoid, and some of its fibers intermingle with the substance of the glenoidal labrum. The tendon curves over the anterior humeral head (Fig. 2.**2**) and enters the intertubercular sulcus (bicipital groove). An extension of the synovial joint space covers the tendon within the groove, and this in turn is covered by the intertubercular ligament (transverse humeral ligament), a short fibrous band roofing the groove.

The teres major is the only intrinsic shoulder muscle which is not a part of the rotator cuff. It originates on the axillary border of the scapula from its lower one-third, below the origin of the teres minor. It extends laterally to the humerus, but unlike the teres minor, crosses in front of the humeral shaft to insert on the medial rim of the intertubercular groove. It thus is primarily an adductor of the humerus and not a rotator muscle. The latissimus dorsi cros-

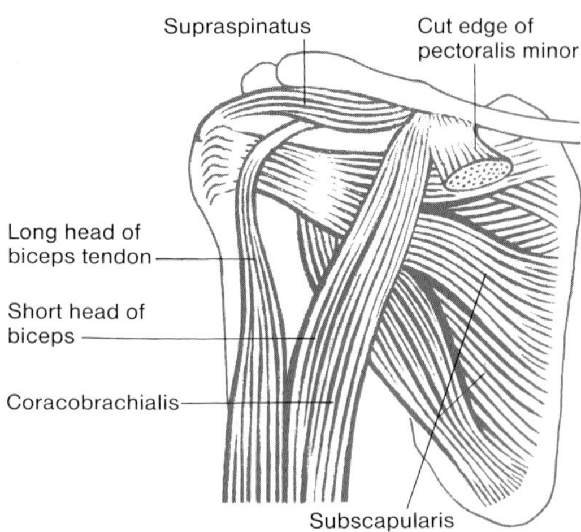

Fig. 2.**2** Anterior view of the deep muscles of the shoulder

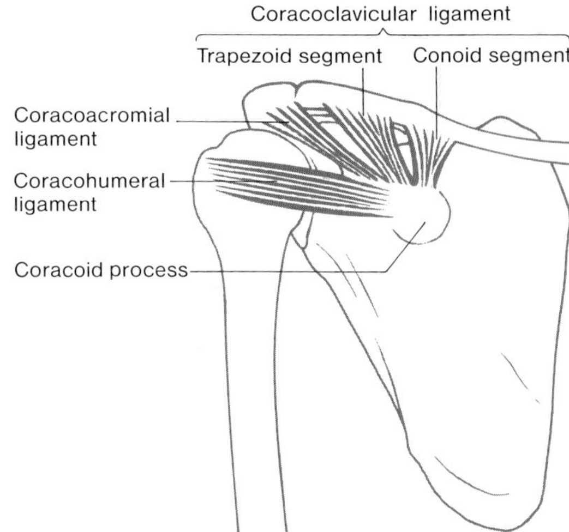

Fig. 2.**3** Anterior view of the ligaments about the shoulder

ses the teres major anteriorly and inserts above the latter on the intertubercular groove.

Other muscles having their origin or insertion on the shoulder will also be seen on MR images in various planes. The most conspicuous of these is the deltoid, originating in a curve extending along the scapular spine, acromion, and clavicle, and covering the outer aspect of the shoulder like a cape (Fig. 2.**1a**). The insertion of the trapezius along the scapu-

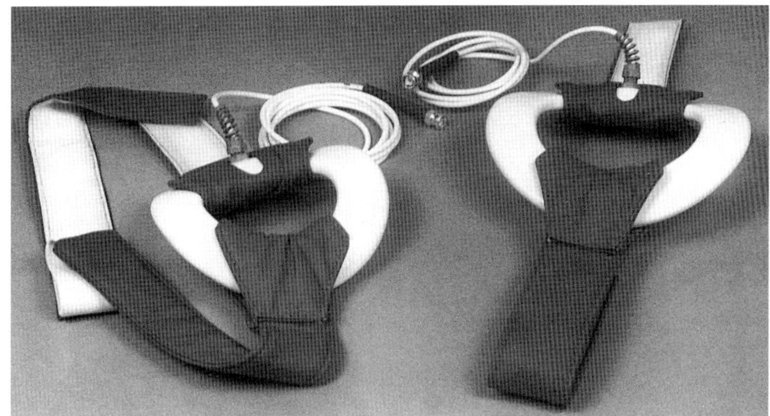

Fig. 2.**4a** Shoulder imaging surface coils of two different sizes (courtesy of Medical Advances, Inc., Milwaukee, Wisconsin)

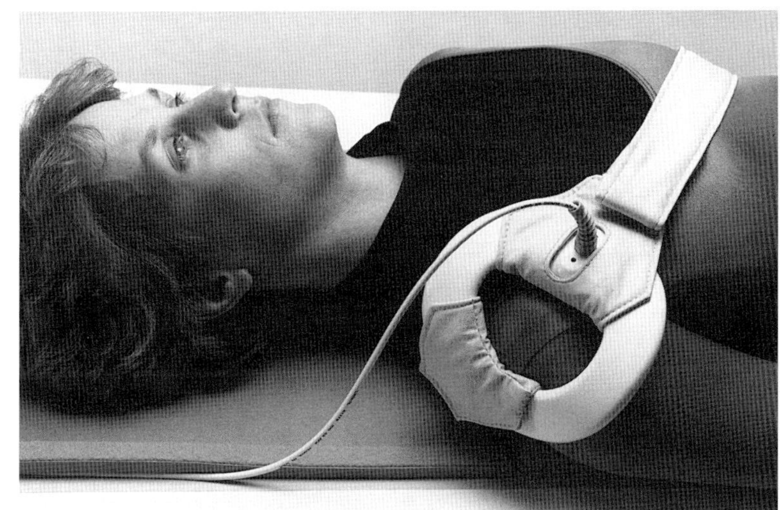

Fig. 2.**4b** The shoulder surface coil is held in place during the MRI procedure by a strap around the patient's chest (courtesy of Medical Advcances, Inc., Milwaukee, Wisconsin)

lar spine, acromion and clavicle will be visible on MR images (Fig. 2.**1a**). The pectoralis minor muscle inserts on the coracoid process, and the coracobrachialis muscle and short head of the biceps muscle of the arm originate on the coracoid process (Fig. 2.**2**). Portions of the pectoralis major, serratus anterior, and triceps muscles will also be observed.

The coracohumeral ligament is situated between the supraspinatus and the subscapularis and also strengthens the capsule anteriorly. Other ligaments helping to stabilize the shoulder are the coracoacromial ligament, which extends obliquely across the anterior and upper aspect of the supraspinatus and which may be a factor in causing shoulder impingement syndrome (see chapter 4), and the coracoclavicular ligament, which is comprised of a trapezoid segment laterally and a conoid segment medially (Fig. 2.**3**).

On MR images, muscle tissue appears with intermediate signal intensity on all sequences. Tendons and cortical bone should appear dark on all sequences. In adults, the bone marrow in the shoulder region is usually fatty and will therefore be white on T1 sequences and progressively less bright on proton density and T2 sequences. If the marrow is still hematogenous, it will produce a gray intermediate signal on all sequences. Subcutaneous fat will have the same appearance as marrow fat. The axillary blood vessels and nerves will be dark.

On the next few pages are examples of images representing portions of three typical imaging sequences. All were obtained on a 1.5 Tesla magnet, and with a shoulder surface coil to receive the signal (Fig. 2.4). The coronal sequence images are oblique to the coronal plane of the body, but parallel to the long axis of the supraspinatus muscle. Each section is 4 mm thick. The TR is 2000 ms and two echoes are recorded at 20 and 60 ms, which will produce, respectively, a proton density–weighted and T2-weighted image for each plane. The field of view is 20 cm. The matrix, or number of individual signals received, is 256 wide by 192 high, for a total of 49152 picture elements making up each image. The scan time is 7 min, 22 s. Between 14 and 20 images (28 to 40 when counting both proton–density and T2-weighted images) are obtained sequentially beginning posteriorly and progressing anteriorly. The axial sequence images are obtained with the same parameters as the coronals, except that there is a 1.5-mm gap between successive axial images and only a 0.5-mm gap between coronals. The sagittal sequence images are T1-weighted with a TE of 20 ms and a TR of 800 ms. Each section is 4 mm thick with a 0.5 mm gap between successive sections. The field of view is 20 cm. The matrix is also 256 by 192. The imaging time is 2 min, 57 s, and 13 images are obtained (Fig. 2.5–7).

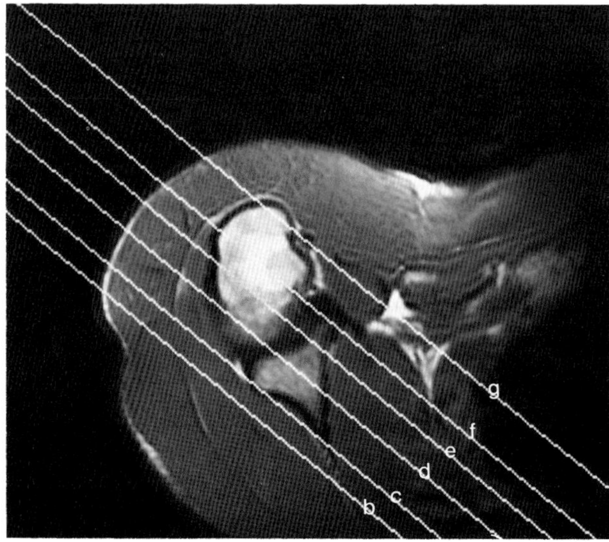

Fig. 2.5 Coronal sections of the shoulder from posterior to anterior. The plane of each section is indicated in **a**, and is parallel to the long axis of the supraspinatus muscle. The images are proton density–weighted

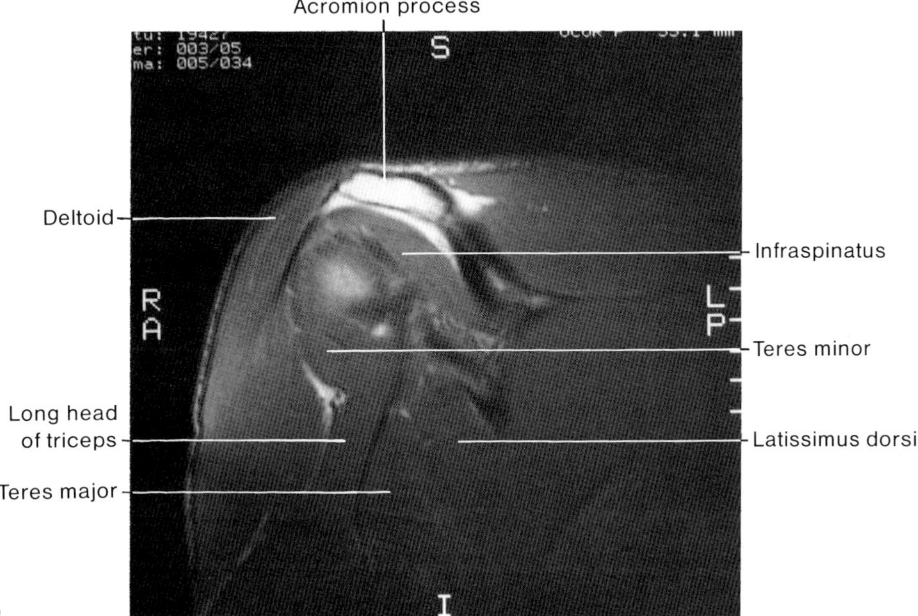

Fig. 2.**5 b**

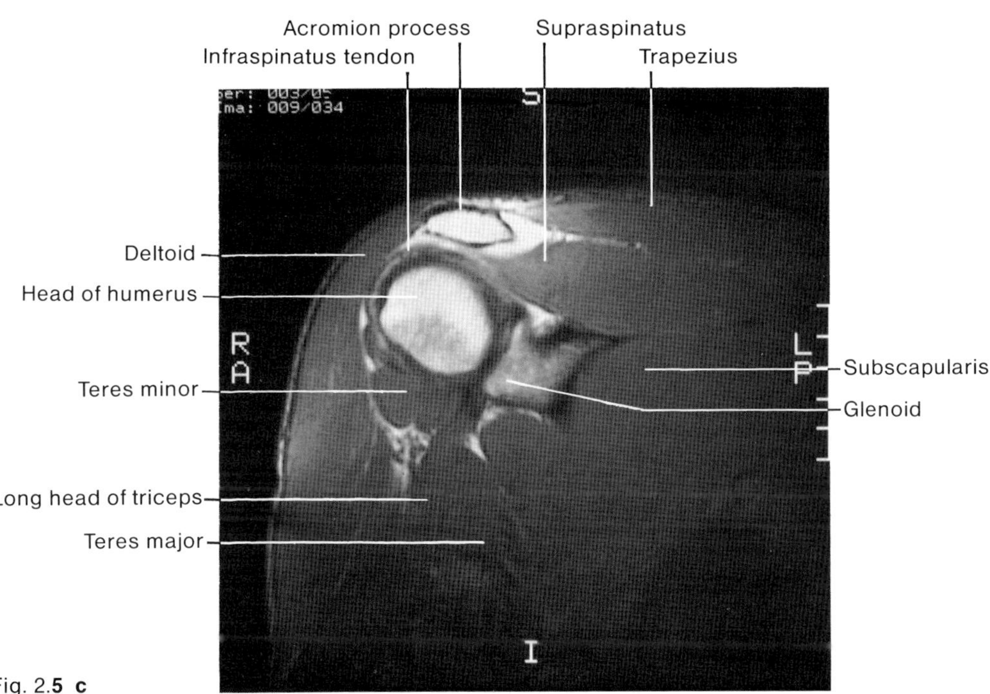

Fig. 2.**5 c**

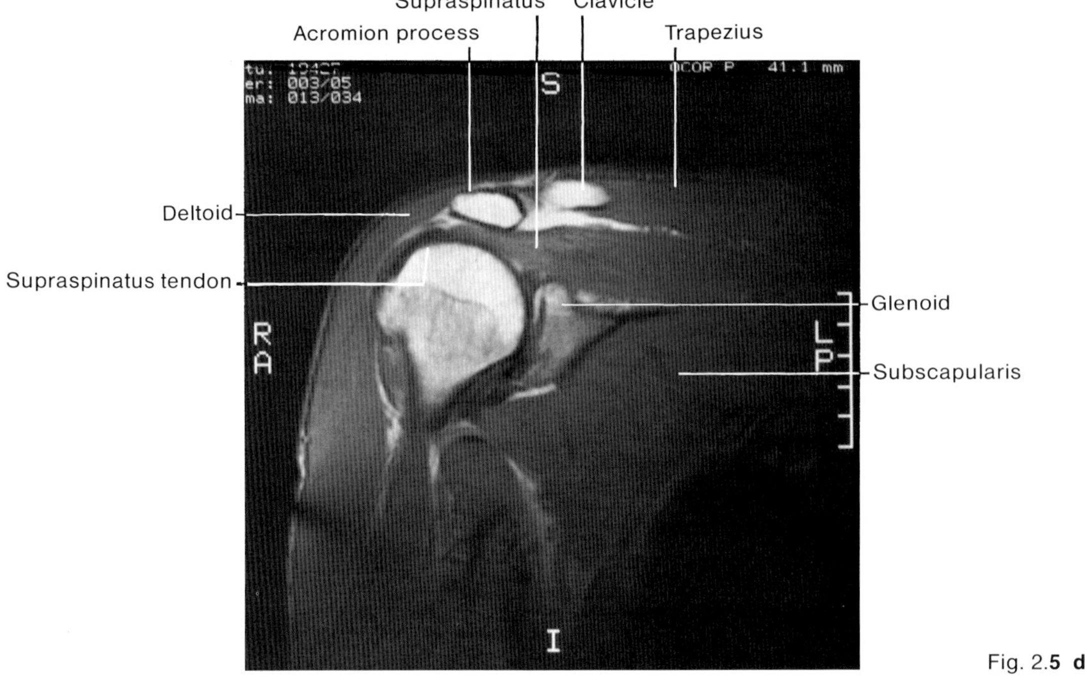

Fig. 2.**5 d**

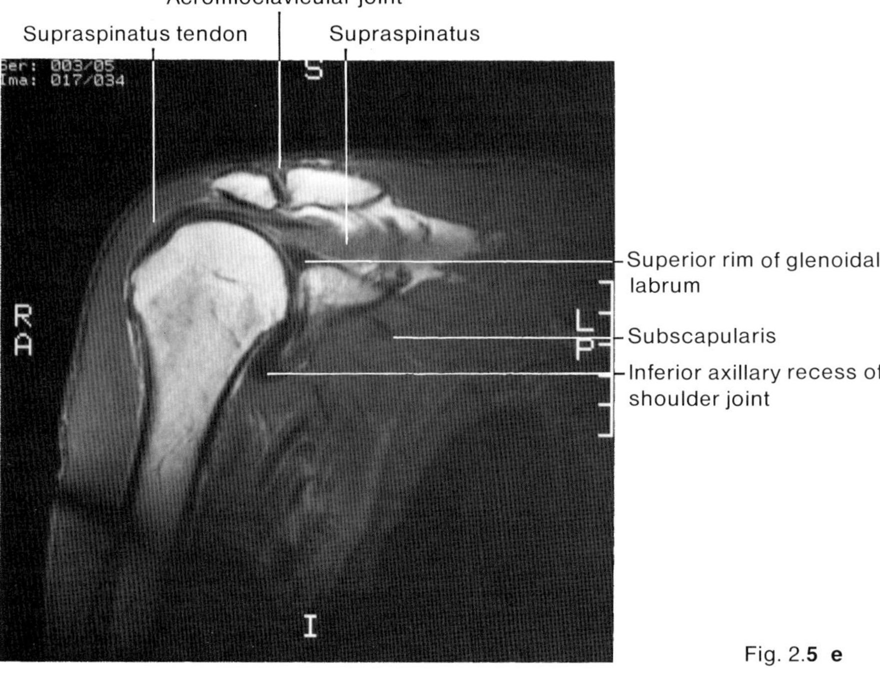

Fig. 2.**5 e**

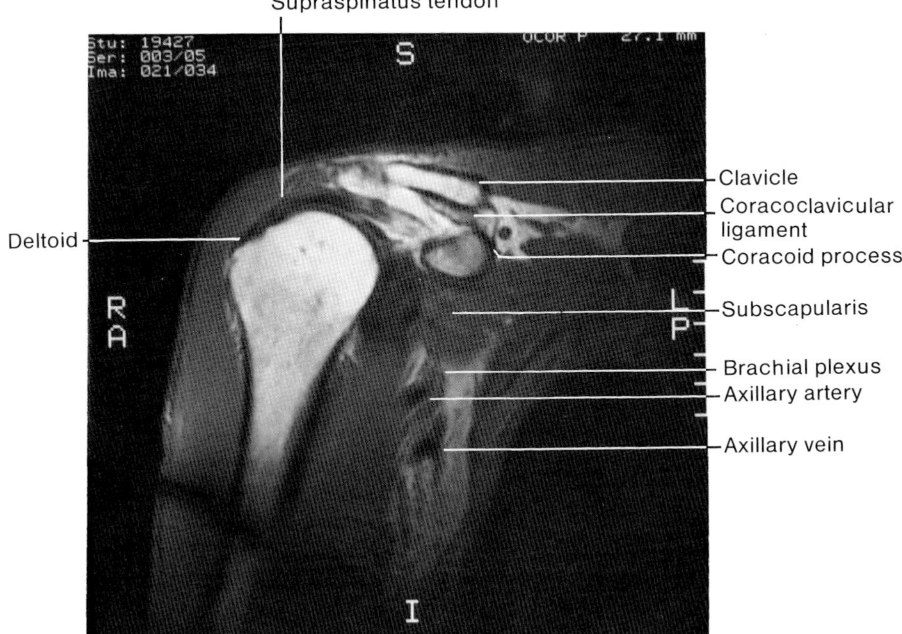

Fig. 2.5 f

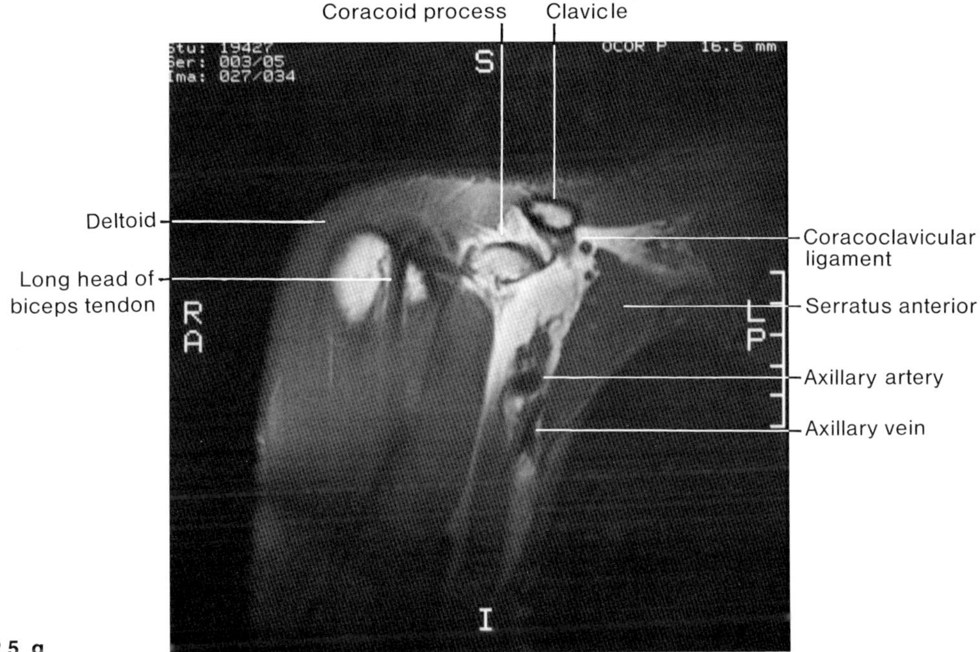

Fig. 2.5 g

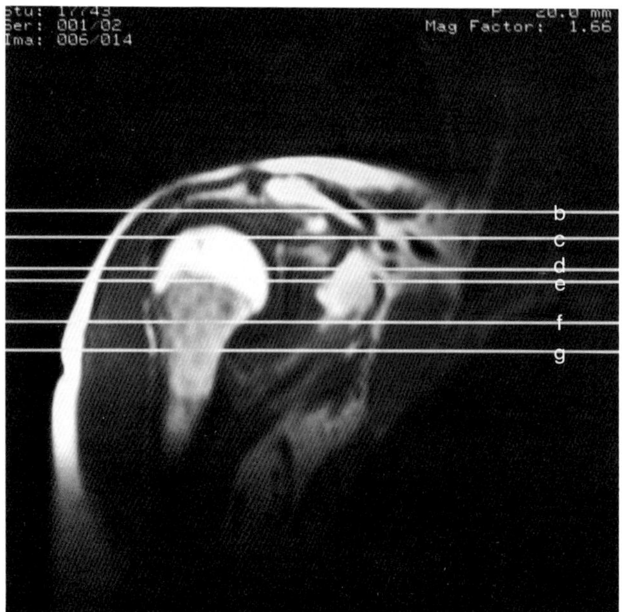

a

Fig. 2.**6**   Axial sections of the shoulder taken from superior to inferior. The plane of each section is shown in **a**. The images are proton density−weighted

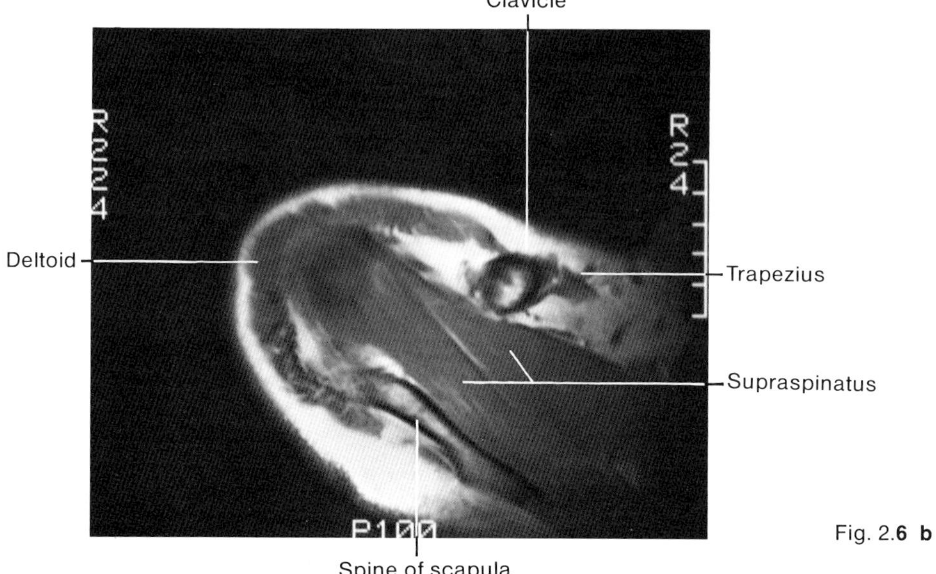

Fig. 2.**6 b**

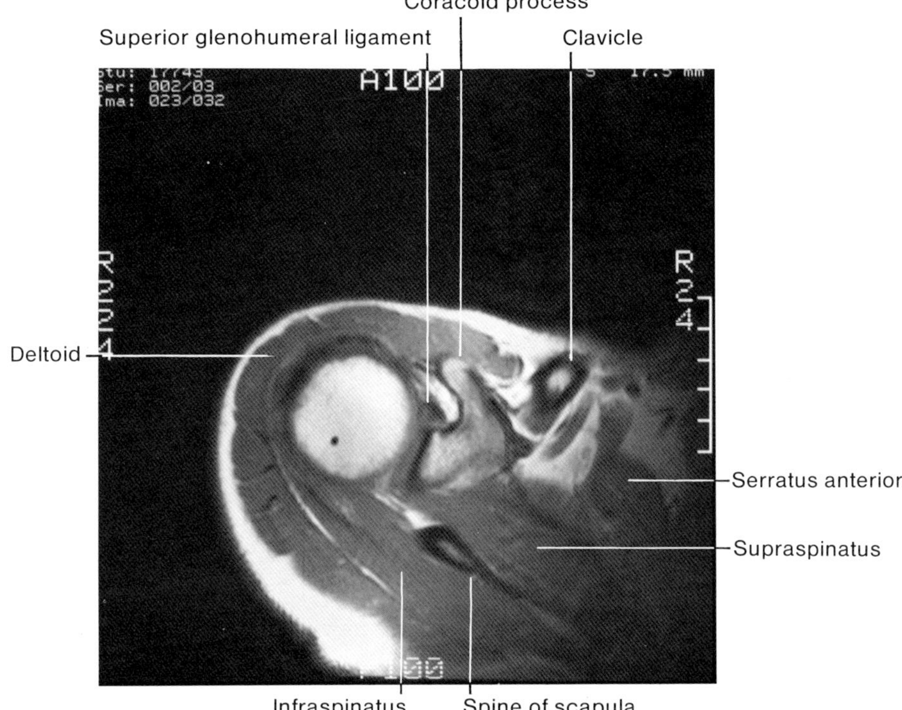

Fig. 2.**6 c**

Fig. 2.**6 d**

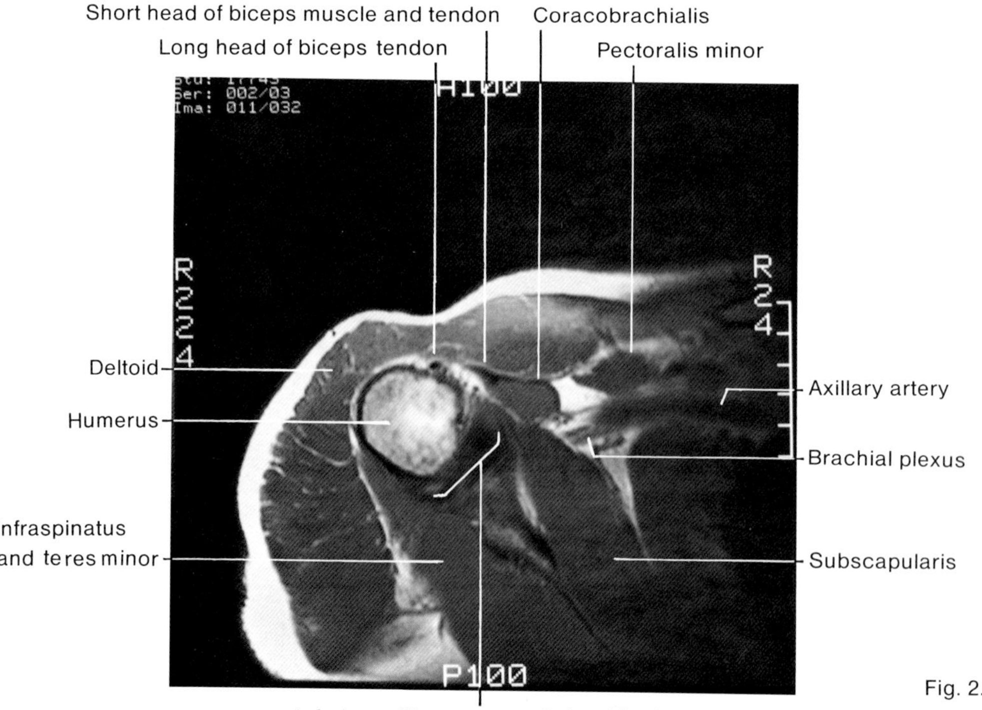

Fig. 2.6 e

Fig. 2.6 f

Short head of biceps
Long head of biceps tendon
Coracobrachialis
Axillary artery
Pectoralis major
Deltoid
Axillary vein
Serratus anterior
Subscapularis
Long head of triceps
Infraspinatus and teres minor

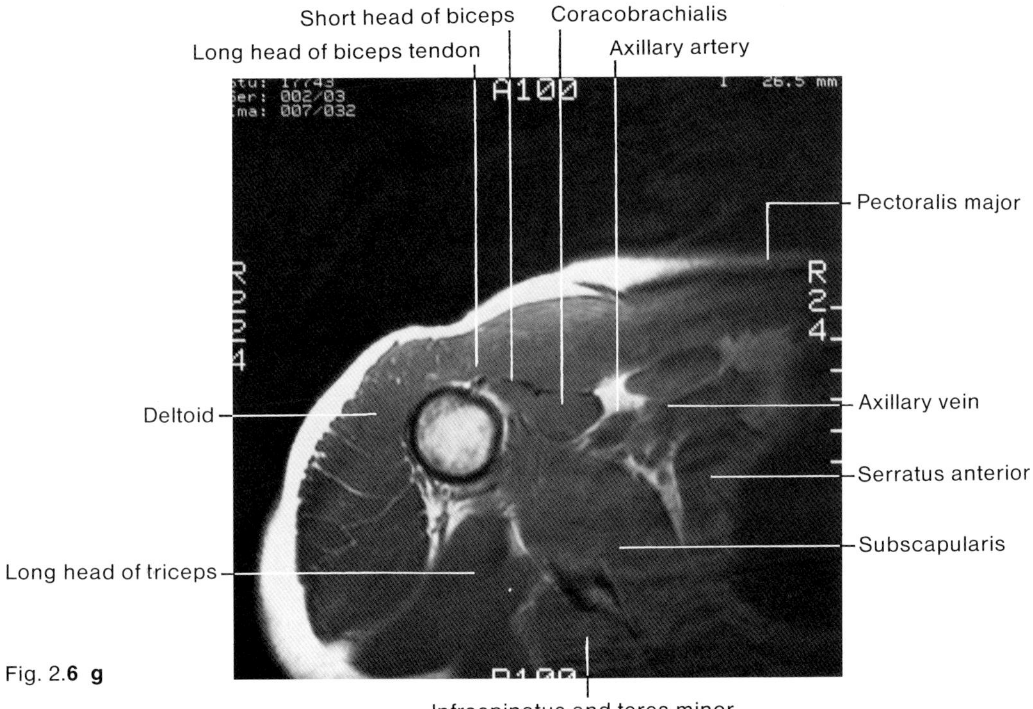

Fig. 2.**6 g**

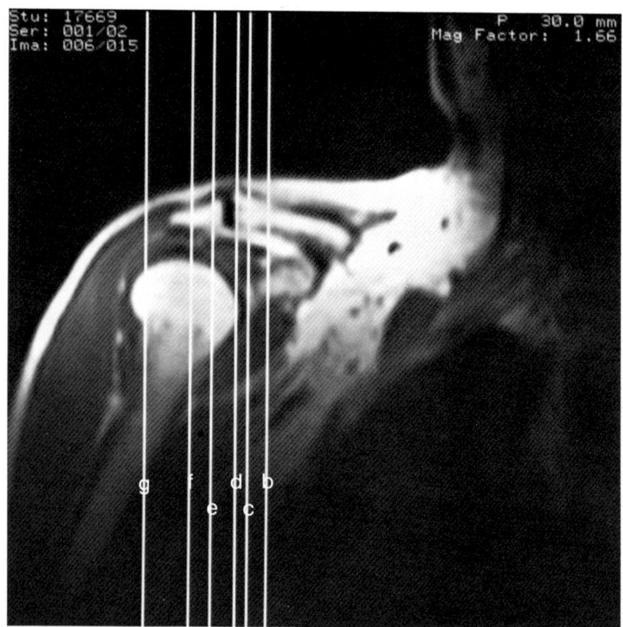

Fig. 2.7   Sagittal sections from medial to lateral. The plane of each section is shown in **a**. The images are T1-weighted

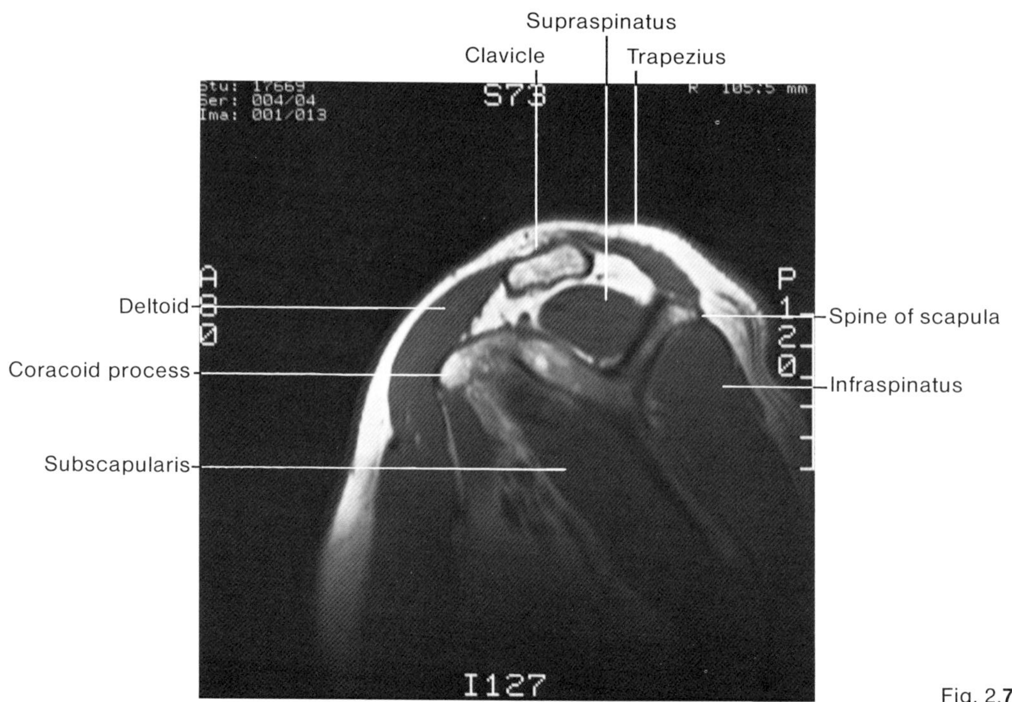

Fig. 2.7 **b**

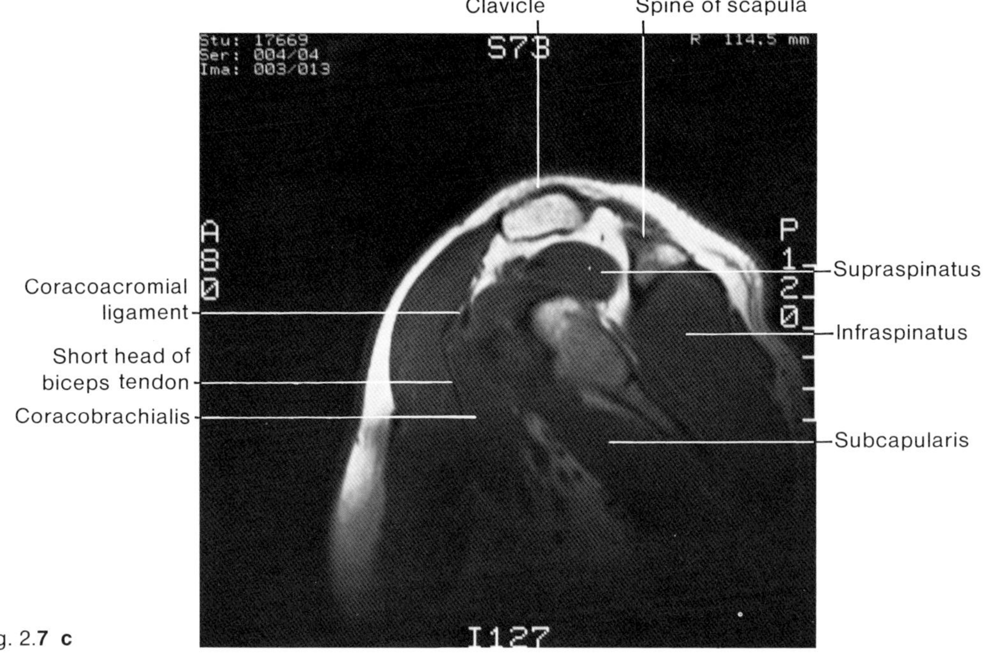

Fig. 2.**7 c**

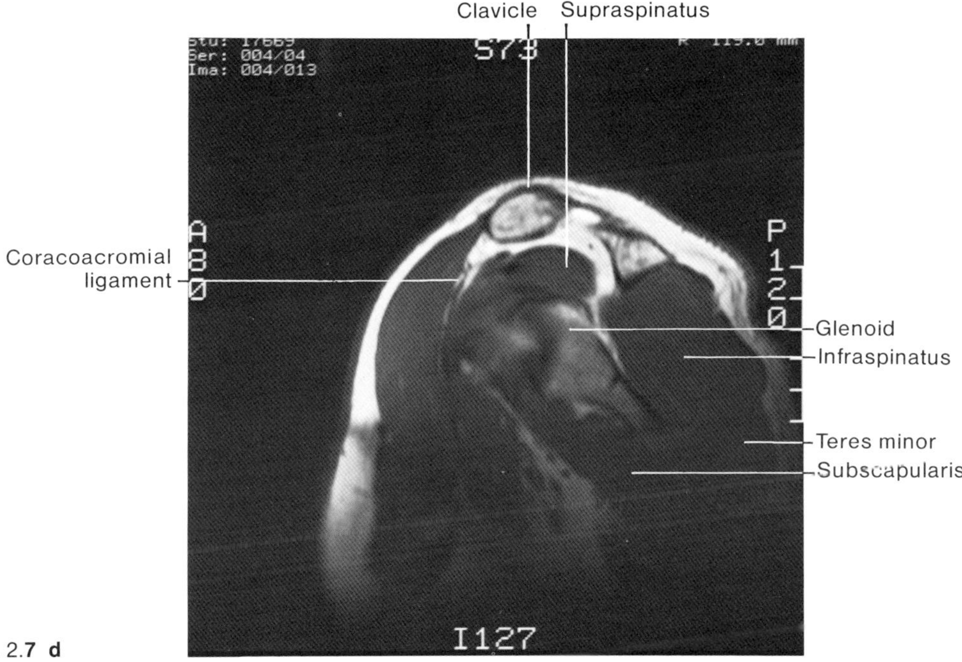

Fig. 2.**7 d**

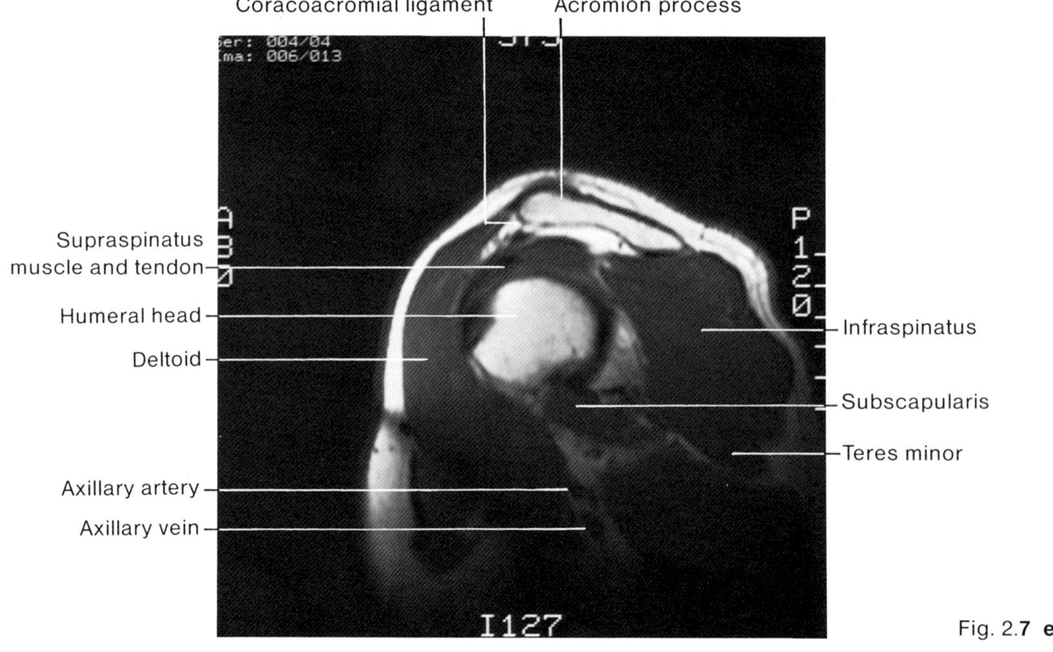

Fig. 2.7 **e**

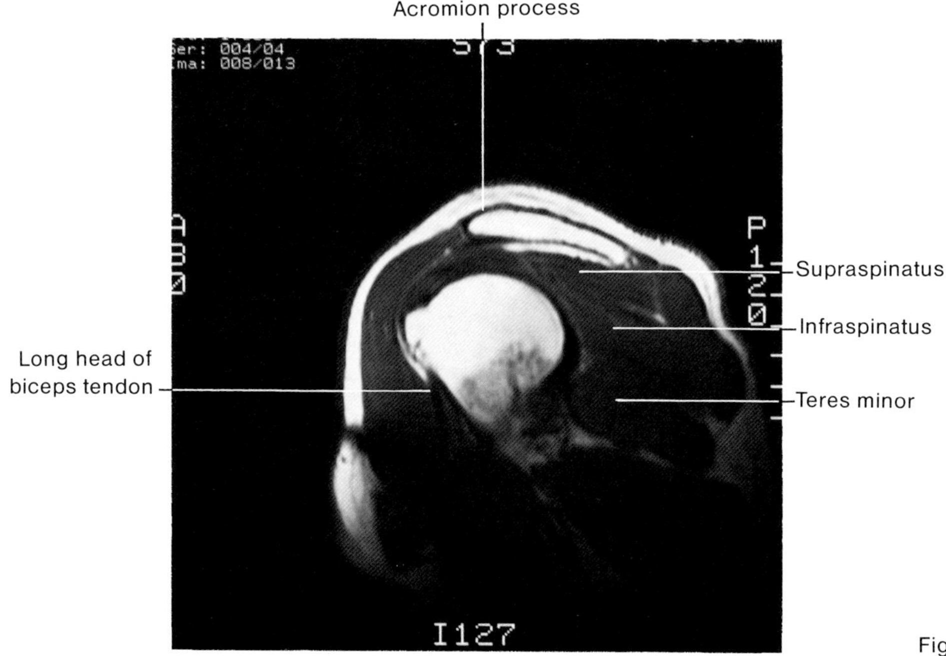

Fig. 2.7 **f**

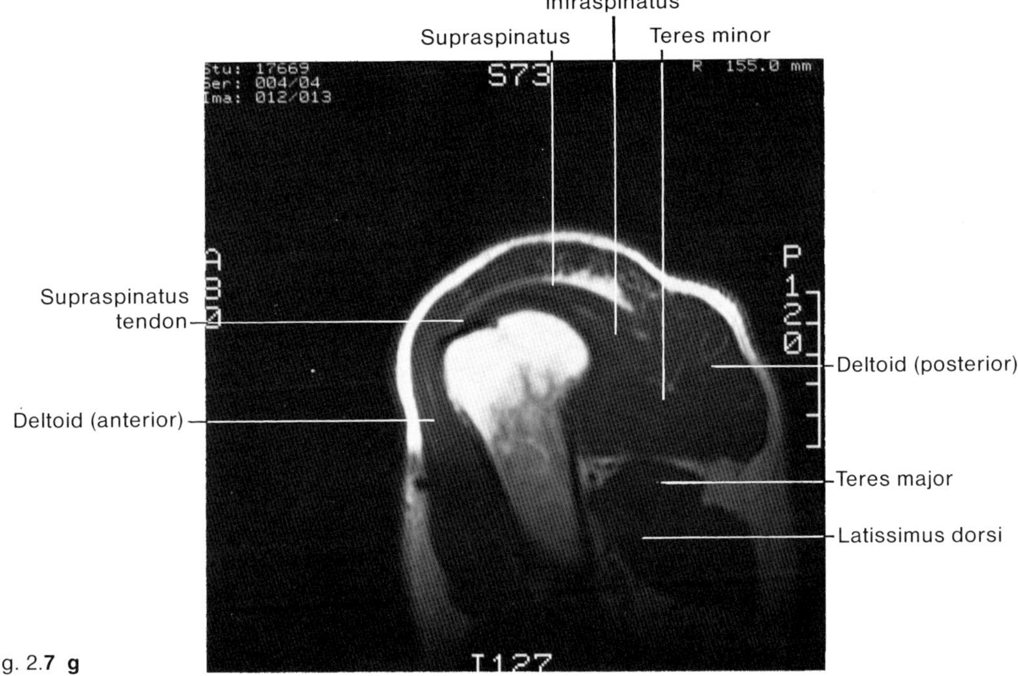

Fig. 2.**7 g**

References

Gray H. Anatomy of the human body. Philadelphia: Lea & Febiger, 1973:454–8.

Kang HS, Resnick D. MRI of the extremities: an anatomic atlas. Philadelphia: WB Saunders, 1991:1–59.

Lockhart RD, Hamilton GF, Fyfe FW. Anatomy of the human body. Philadelphia: JB, Lippencott, 1959:197–211.

Middleton WD, Lawson TL. Anatomy and MRI of the joints. New York: Raven Press, 1989:13–48.

3 Diagnosis of Shoulder Disorders

The evaluation of shoulder pathology is difficult due to the proximity of neurovascular and musculotendinous structures about this articulation. A basic knowledge of the complex anatomy of this area is essentiel in order to formulate an opinion as to the possible diagnoses of disorders in this area.

A thorough *patient history* should be taken prior to evaluating the patient since it allows the physician to perform a more efficient physical examination. The examiner should begin the evaluation by noting the patient's age and dominant extremity. Although overhead lifting requires use of both upper extremities and may result in injuries to either shoulder, throwing athletes are obviously more prone to injury in their dominant extremity. Cervical disorders may present with shoulder pain.

The onset of injury should also be determined. Some patients have sustained a major trauma while others will report that they had an insidious onset of symptoms. Acute trauma is often responsible for dislocations or fractures of the shoulder. Dislocations of the glenohumeral joint are usually anterior and are common in contact sports (Rockwood and Green, 1984). In cases of recurrent instability, the frequency of dislocation should be noted. Posterior dislocations are less common, and often are due to falls on an outstretched arm (Rockwood and Green, 1984). Acromioclavicular separations are often due to falls onto the shoulder. If the patient has any radiographs which were obtained at the time of the injury, he or she should bring them. They will help determine the direction of instability, as it is often impossible to evaluate the acutely injured patient because of his or her pain. Patients frequently relate that they "dislocated" their glenohumeral joint, when, in fact, they have suffered acromioclavicular separations.

Many injuries, however, do not involve acute trauma and these patients are often unable to cite an injury associated with their disabilities. They will often have attempted to treat themselves with various "home remedies" and inadequate doses of over-the-counter medications. Pain that persists in spite of adequate dosage may indicate significant pathology. Some patients may be referred by other physicians and may have had injections in the past. The type, frequency and location of injections should be noted.

The type and location of pain is also important. Pain of cervical origin may be a radicular or burning type of pain, while rotator cuff injuries may present with dull, aching pain. Some patients complain of pain when they sleep on the affected shoulder. This may indicate advanced pathology. The extent to which this pain affects the patient's daily life should also be determined. Pain may occur only when the patient is involved in strenuous activities, whereas others complain of a pain that affects the activities of daily living.

The location of pain may be helpful in determining whether the patient has primary shoulder or cervical pathology. Cervical involvement typically produces pain along the superior aspect of the shoulder and in the interscapular region. Patients with posterior shoulder pain due to levator scapulae syndrome will localize the pain to its insertion on the scapula.

Pain on the superior aspect of the shoulder may indicate pathology of the acromioclavicular joint. These patients often are able to localize the acromioclavicular joint as the source of their pain and many present with a history of trauma.

Patients with rotator cuff pathology often present with pain in the area of the deltoid, often indicating the deltoid insertion as the source of their discomfort. Some of these patients present after having had "trigger point" injections at the deltoid tuberosity.

Bicipital tendinitis and anterior instability may both present with anterior shoulder discomfort. Pain due to instability may also be accompanied by a catching sensation if there are associated labrum tears or loose bodies. Posterior shoulder pain may be seen in patients with posterior instability, or may occur with anterior instability due to traction on the posterior capsule.

Degenerative arthritis presents with multifocal pain.

Lesions of the brachial plexus, such as brachial neuritis, may also present with anterior shoulder pain. Less common are neurovascular disorders, such as thoracic outlet syndrome. This diagnosis should be made carefully, only after excluding all other possible diagnoses, since objective tests may not be helpful in supporting this diagnosis (Rockwood and Matsen, 1990). Vascular studies should be performed in patients who demonstrate asymmetrical diminution or loss of pulses in the upper extremity. The presence of a cervical rib on routine chest radiographs may also suggest that this may be a source of the patient's disability (Rockwood and Matsen, 1990).

The patient's overall health should also be determined. Systemic disorders, such as diabetes mellitus, may be associated with adhesive capsulitis. Patients with tumors which metastasize to bone may require further diagnostic tests if shoulder involvement is suspected. Young patients may present with pathologic fractures or shoulder pain due to primary bone tumors. Stress fractures of the proximal humeral physis may occur in Little League pitchers.

Age may be helpful in formulating a diagnosis since shoulder disorders occur most frequently in older patients. One should not assume, however, that significant injuries cannot occur in younger patients. Athletes now begin training at very early ages and may present with advanced lesions due to overuse injuries. Often, patients will be referred to a specialist with the preliminary diagnosis of a shoulder sprain, when, in fact, they may have advanced evidence of instability or rotator cuff pathology.

Physical examination of the shoulder begins with observation of the patient's posture. Patients who participate in overhead sports may present with depression of the dominant shoulder due to elongation of the scapular rotators.

Other patients with significant shoulder pain may hold the painful shoulder in an elevated position. It is helpful to observe the patient's gait pattern to determine whether they swing their arms comfortably when they walk. The patient should also be observed performing activities of daily life, such as putting on a shirt or reaching up to comb his or her hair. Patients with cervical pain may avoid excessive motion of their heads to avoid pain.

The shoulder should be inspected for atrophy, such as that which may be seen with suprascapular neuropathy or rotator cuff tears. Muscular wasting of the affected limb may indicate the presence of a nerve injury. A distally retracted biceps tear may be seen with impingement lesions and may be noted on examining the arm.

The initial inspection is followed by an evaluation of the patient's motion. The point at which pain begins should be documented since some patients with moderate pain tolerance may demonstrate excellent but painful motion.

The Society of American Shoulder and Elbow Surgeons recommends measurement of total elevation, external rotation with the arm at the side and at 90° of abduction, and internal rotation (Rockwood and Matsen, 1990). Total elevation is performed by elevating the shoulder to 20°–30° from the sagittal plane and is measured on the lateral view. Passive external rotation should be measured with the patient supine. Loss of active and/or passive external rotation may indicate rotator cuff pathology, which also may be accompanied by painful abduction. These patients may also present with painful forward flexion. Loss of active external rotation due to apprehension may also be seen in patients with anterior instability, particularly when the arm is simultaneously abducted beyond 90°. Excessive passive external rotation may be seen in athletes who participate heavily in overhead sports; it develops as an adaption to the repetitive external rotation needed for these activities. Pain along the superior aspect of the shoulder that arises with attempts to bring the arm across the chest to touch the posterior aspect of the unaffected shoulder may indicate pathology of the acromioclavicular joint.

When observing active motion, the examiner should also determine if there are any compensatory motions, such as scapulothoracic substitution, which may occur with rotator cuff pathology. Scapular winging may be noted with palsy of the long thoracic nerve.

Severe restriction in motion may occur with massive rotator cuff tears or in some patients who have very painful partial tears. Capsulitis may also be associated with a significant loss of motion. The extent of the loss of motion can only be determined by comparison with the patient's unaffected extremity, since there is significant patient-to-patient variability.

Tenderness in various structures when palpated is also an important component of the physical examination. The examination begins systematically with palpation of the cervical and paracervical structures, particularly in patients who have a history which would make one suspect cervical disease.

The acromioclavicular joint is a common area of tenderness, particularly in older patients with impingement. The repetitive activity that is associated with degenerative rotator cuff disease in these patients may also lead to degenerative changes in the acromioclavicular joint. This commonly involves loss of the acromioclavicular joint space and osteophyte formation of the inferior distal clavicle and the adjacent inferior edge of the anterior acromion. Osteophytes which project inferiorly into the subacromial space further compromise the size of this space. This leads to further impingement on the rotator cuff in these patients. Any patient who complains of impingement-type symptoms should therefore be examined carefully to also evaluate the acromioclavicular joint.

Gross deformity of this joint may be present in patients who have sustained major trauma to this area, such as acromioclavicular separations. Direct tenderness of the distal clavicle may also occur with osteolysis in some athletes (Cahill, 1982).

Impingement pain is commonly felt in the area associated with the most common area of rotator cuff injury, the insertion of the supraspinatus tendon (Rathbun and McNab, 1970). This is most easily palpated at the anterolateral border of the acromion. The anterior border of the acromion is also a common point of tenderness, since subacromial osteophytes and the coracoacromial ligament, structures which are thought to contribute to subacromial impingement, are located in this area.

Another area of potential tenderness is the bicipital groove, where the long head of the biceps can be palpated. Injuries to this structure may accompany degenerative changes of the rotator cuff. Dislocation of the tendon from the bicipital groove may occur with complete rotator cuff tears. Isolated dislocation of the bicipital tendon, due to a hypoplastic bicipital groove, may also occur.

Anterior shoulder tenderness may also be observed in patients with anterior shoulder instability and associated injuries to the anterior capsule, and brachial plexus neuritis. Comparison with the unaffected shoulder should be performed, however, since deep palpation in this area may elicit pain simply to the pressure applied during the examination.

Posterior capsular tenderness may be seen in patients with instability or in patients with injuries to the posterior rotator cuff.

Maneuvers which are designed to elicit pain, such as resistive testing of selected muscle groups about the shoulder are also helpful. The most useful tests for rotator cuff pathology involve resisted abduction of the involved extremity with the arm in maximal internal rotation, and resisted external rotation (Figs. 3.1, 3.2). Pain with resisted flexion of the arm, as well resisted supination of the fore-

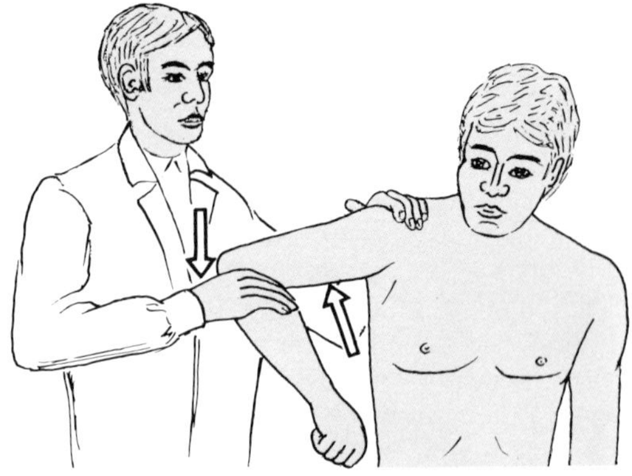

Fig. 3.1 Pain with resisted abduction in maximal internal rotation may indicate pathology of the rotator cuff

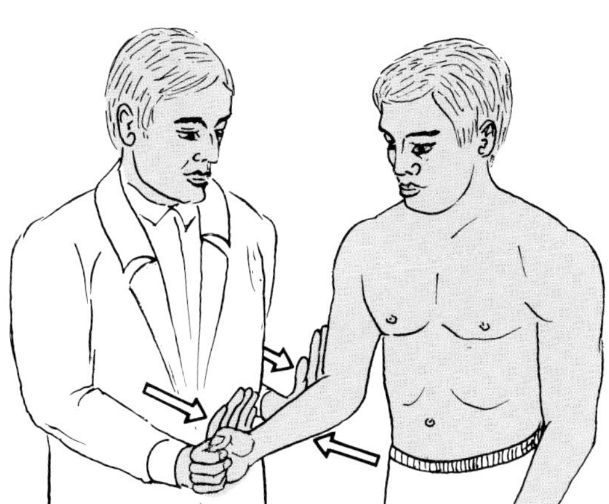

Fig. 3.**2** Testing resisted external rotation. If painful, this may indicate pathology of the rotator cuff

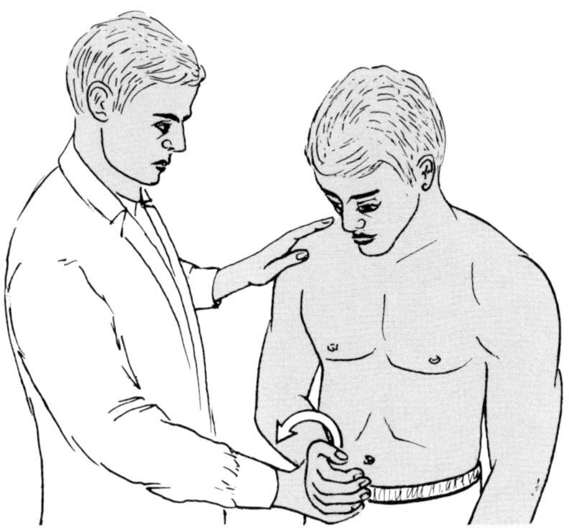

Fig. 3.**3** Resisted supination of the forearm may elicit bicipital pain

arm, may be noted in the bicipital groove, and may indicate pathology of the tendon of the long head of the biceps (Fig. 3.**3**).

Resistive testing should be performed on all major muscle groups of the shoulder to detect any associated pain or weakness. The cervical spine and the arm musculature should also be evaluated. Weakness with resistive testing may be due to a neurologic injury and may be accompanied by loss of sensation. Further objective tests, such as nerve conduction studies or an EMG may be necessary.

Suprascapular neuropathy may occur with compression of the nerve at the scapular notch by the transverse scapular ligament. Axillary nerve injury may accompany anterior dislocations of the glenohumeral joint. This may not be appreciated initially due to the pain and disability which accompanies the dislocation. Sensory examination of the epaulet area of the shoulder will often reveal decreased sensation with axillary nerve injuries. Injuries to the long thoracic nerves may also not be detected easily unless the serratus anterior strength is evaluated separately.

Crepitation with movement of the shoulder may also be noted during the evaluation, although its clinical significance may vary. The crepitation may be due to scapulothoracic pathology, such as an exostosis on the deep surface of the scapula, degenerative changes in

the acromioclavicular joint, or subacromial bursitis. The source can normally be determined by physical examination, and may or may not require treatment. Many patients show great concern about this crepitation and require assurance if it is thought to be nonpathologic. Painful crepitation, such as that which may occur with rotator cuff tears, requires further evaluation of the underlying structures. Crepitation may also be due to sternoclavicular joint injuries and this should be evaluated in patients with an appropriate history.

Provocative tests designed to elicit instability in patients with an appropriate history should be performed routinely. The most common test is the "apprehension test" performed in the upright position and which, when positive, suggests anterior or anterior inferior instability (Fig. 3.**4**). This test should elicit true apprehension on the patient's part and is best performed so that one can evaluate the patient's facial expression and lack of muscle relaxation due to the feeling of impending dislocation. It is also helpful to have the patient actively externally rotate the humerus at 90° of abduction prior to performing the apprehension test. If the patient is apprehensive in this position, it should alert the examiner to perform the test gently.

Pain with the apprehension test is not neces-

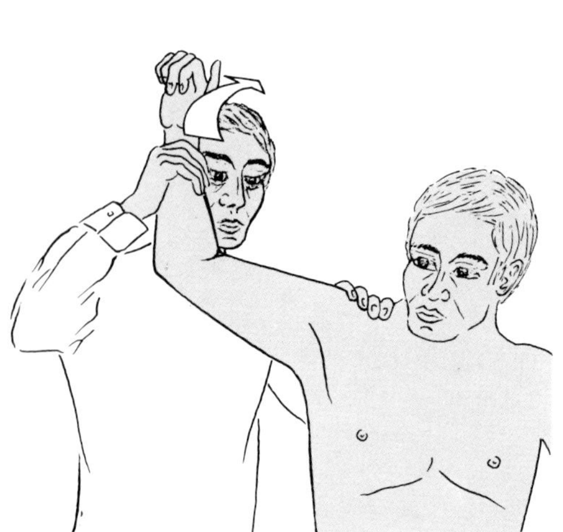

Fig. 3.**4** The apprehension test in the upright position is seen here. Pain during this maneuver may be due to impingement

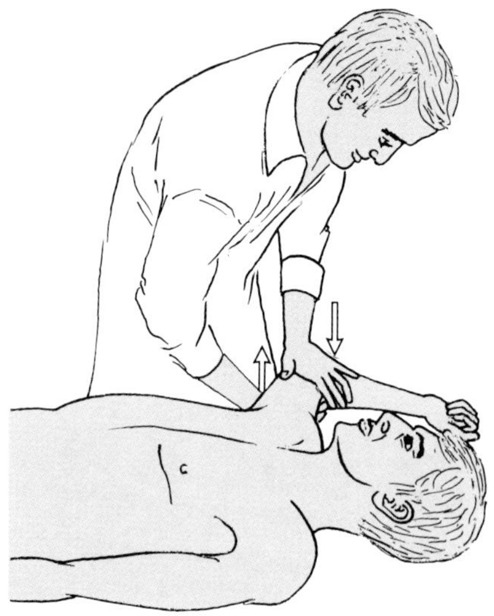

Fig. 3.**5** The apprehension test in the supine position. This helps eliminate pain due to impingement

sarily indicative of instability and may be due, instead, to impingement of the rotator cuff. This has led to a modification of the apprehension test, which involves examination of the patient in the supine position (Fig. 3.**5**). This eliminates the pain due to impingement of the rotator cuff which may occur in the hyperabducted and externally rotated positions. The supine test also allows the examiner to evaluate the amount of translation of the glenohumeral joint in patients in whom instability is suspected.

Posterior instability may be more subtle and difficult to detect. Posterior translation should be evaluated in the upright and supine positions. These patients may demonstrate apprehension as they bring their arm across the chest in a position of maximal internal rotation, and then elevate the limb. Some patients may be able to actively subluxate or dislocate posteriorly. These patients often demonstrate abnormal excessive activity in the anterior deltoid at the expense of a weaker posterior deltoid. Surgical procedures for posterior instability do not have high success rates such as those seen with treatment of anterior instability. Conservative treatment is indicated for most

of these patients, particularly with posterior instability that is nontraumatic or voluntary.

Inferior instability is less common and may be noted in patients who demonstrate generalized hyperelasticity of the soft tissues. The examiner may be able to passively subluxate the glenohumeral joint with traction distally on the affected arm. "Dimpling" at the lateral border of the acromion, which occurs when the shoulder subluxates inferiorly, may be noted. These patients also have been shown to respond poorly to soft-tissue procedures, but may require surgical treatment if prolonged conservative treatment fails.

Recently, authors such as Jobe have proposed that anterior instability and impingement may occur simultaneously (1989). It has long been known that older patients who dislocate their shoulders often have associated tears of the rotator cuff. This is probably due to a traction injury of the rotator cuff as it attempts to keep the humeral head reduced during the dislocation episode. The most important static stabilizer preventing anterior dislocation in most instances is the inferior glenohumeral ligament. Athletes with both anterior instability and impingement are thought to have impingement due to the excessive anterior translation. Treatment of the impingement alone in these patients will probably not correct the patients' disability since the primary lesion is one of instability.

Other possible injuries in athletes who participate in overhead sports are injuries to the posterior rotator cuff, thought to be due to deceleration injuries in the follow-through stage of the throwing motion. Patients may complain of pain when the posterior glenohumeral joint and the posterior rotator cuff, which is in intimate contact with the posterior capsule, are palpated.

Another possible deceleration injury is a traumatic detachment of the superior labrum, the SLAP lesion which is the site of attachment of the long head of the biceps to the labrum. This tendon is thought to be a stabilizer of the glenohumeral joint as well. Injuries to this complex may produce anterior shoulder pain, and pain may be elicited with resistive testing of the biceps (Fig. 3.**3**).

Objective tests of shoulder pathology have undergone a tremendous change over the past few years. Plain radiographs can yield important information about the extent of degenerative changes such as those of the glenohumeral and acromioclavicular joints. Dislocations of the acromioclavicular joints or the glenohumeral joint may be seen easily with plain radiographs. The extent of instability or dislocation may not be appreciated without the use of weights in some patients. The weights should be suspended from the wrists, not grasped. These views can be used not only for the acromioclavicular joint, but also for inferior or multidirectional instability, which may produce inferior subluxation of the humeral head from the glenoid on AP radiographs. The supraspinatus outlet view allows evaluation of the inferior anterior acromial surface, which may compromise the subacromial space in patients with impingement lesions.

Skeletally immature patients pose a special problem with regard to radiographic evaluation of the shoulder. The presence of open physes in these patients makes evaluation of radiographs difficult. Comparison views should be routinely obtained in this age group. This is particularly useful in patients with pos-

sible stress injuries of the proximal humeral physis, which may cause a widening of the physis.

Arthrograms using contrast material are useful for detecting complete rotator cuff tears, although visualizing partial tears may be difficult. Extravasation of contrast material or air into the subacromial space is the hallmark of complete rotator cuff tears.

Computed tomography is useful in some patients in whom a bony lesion is suspected, such as a Bankart lesion with a fracture or erosion of the anterior glenoid. This test may also demonstrate evidence of humeral head changes associated with dislocations. The Hill–Sachs defect is an indentation fracture of the posterior humeral head which may occur with anterior dislocations. Anterior head indentation fractures, the reverse Hill–Sachs defect, may be seen with posterior shoulder dislocations. Patients with recurrent posterior dislocations may also demonstrate an abnormal glenoid tilt which predisposes the patient to posterior dislocation. This may be determined by evaluating the glenoid surfaces on the CT scans.

CT arthrograms are also useful, particularly with patients in whom a labrum defect is suspected, such as with dislocations of the glenohumeral joint. Excessive capsular laxity may also be demonstrated with these tests.

Fluoroscopic evaluation of the patient under anesthesia may also be necessary in select cases. Evaluation of the uninvolved shoulder should always be performed.

Ultrasonography has been used to demonstrate rotator cuff pathology. Its main advantage is that it is noninvasive. Evaluation of the results of this test, however, is difficult, and the accuracy of the result depends on the evaluator.

The advent of magnetic resonance imaging has been particularly helpful for patients with partial rotator cuff tears or tendinitis in whom arthrograms or ultrasound may not be diagnostic. The rotator cuff can be evaluated in multiple views and the extent of a tear determined. This is useful in planning operative procedures since the amount or retraction and the size of the tear may help determine the type of procedure chosen. Degenerative changes, both in the glenohumeral and the acromioclavicular joints, and subacromial impingement may also be assessed. The bicipital groove and its tendon can be easily visualized. Fluid accumulation in its tendon sheath may be seen with tendinitis. Bone disorders, such as avascular necrosis or tumors, and synovial disorders, such as synovial chondromatosis, can be diagnosed. MRI is safer than plain radiographs since there is no radiation exposure, but some patients feel claustrophobic in the MRI machine and require premedication.

Injections may be used to verify and treat a diagnosis made during the physical examination of a patient. The material injected is commonly a mixture of a local anesthetic and an anti-inflammatory medication, and is used most often in the subacromial space and the acromioclavicular joint. Injections of the bicipital tendon should be done infrequently and carefully since it may precipitate rupture of the tendon.

The diagnosis of shoulder disorders, therefore, begins with a careful history, which helps determine which part of the physical examination needs special emphasis. Objective tests, such as MRI, should be used to substantiate a provisional diagnosis but do not need to be obtained in all patients. They are helpful, however, in preoperative planning for patients requiring surgery.

References

Cahill BR. Osteolysis of the distal part of the clavicle in male athletes. J Bone Joint Surg 1982; 64A(7):1053–8.
Jobe FW. Instructional course lectures, vol. 38. AAOS, 1989.
Rockwood CR, Green DR. Fractures in adults. Philadelphia: JB Lippincott, 1984.
Rockwood CR, Matsen FA. The shoulder. Philadelphia: WB Saunders, 1990.
Rathbun JB, McNab I. The microvascular pattern of the rotator cuff. J Bone Joint Surg 1970; 52B(3):540–53.

4 Magnetic Resonance Imaging of Patients with Shoulder Pain or Instability

The muscles of the rotator cuff and their tendons envelop the humeral head and attach to the greater and lesser tuberosities. Their fasciae blend with the shoulder joint capsule. These are the muscles of internal and external shoulder rotation. An injury to the rotator cuff is a frequently seen cause of disability. The injury can involve any or all of the muscles or their tendons. In fact, however, the supraspinatus and its tendon are by far the most commonly involved.

The supraspinatus initiates abduction of the arm. It extends from the supraspinatus fossa of the scapula over the upper glenohumeral joint capsule and inserts on the uppermost of three tubercles of the greater tuberosity. The lateral muscle fibers, the musculotendinous junction, and the tendon are sandwiched between the acromion and acromioclavicular joint above and the humeral head below. The subacromial bursa is situated between the muscle and the acromion and cushions the stress caused by continual friction of motion on the bone. With the arm in the neutral position, the lateral supraspinatus fibers and the musculotendinous junction lie anterior to the acromion. With flexion of the humerus, the anterior portion of the supraspinatus tendon moves superiorly (Fig. 4.1). Degenerative changes occur on the acromion with the formation of bony spurs. If the spurs are directed inferiorly, the result is a compromised space between the acromion and the humeral head, and compression of the supraspinatus.

It has been shown that the critical area of supraspinatus impingement is on the anterior aspect of the acromion process (Neer and Welsh, 1977). Friction and wear on the tendon occur as the muscle contracts and the arm is abducted. This is one cause of the *shoulder impingement syndrome.*

As the arm is elevated above the horizontal, the tendon is drawn medially and slides under the acromioclavicular joint. The coracoacromial ligament extends across the anterior region of the tendon and musculotendinous junction of the supraspinatus.

Imaging of the shoulder with the arm at the side cannot demonstrate the impingement that occurs with the arm elavated. With current technology, MR scanners keep the patient confined during the examination, preventing them from assuming the position of maximal shoulder impingement during imaging. Furthermore, an MR sequence can last from 6 to 10 min for each body plane being imaged, a length of time for which the patient could not be expected to assume the position of greatest discomfort. Therefore, very early changes of bony impingement on the rotator cuff may not be apparent on an MR image and require clinical evaluation for diagnosis.

There is no absolute measurement of the space between the acromion and humeral head which distinguishes a normal state from shoulder impingement. The humerus can be voluntarily drooped, allowing ample room for the rotator cuff, in someone who may have severe shoulder impingement when the arm is in the

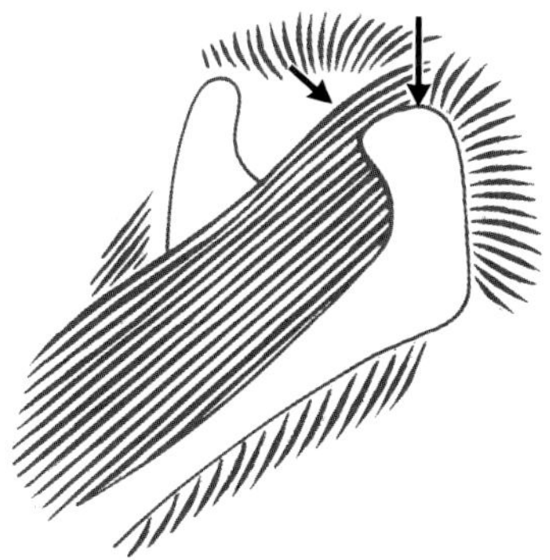

Fig. 4.1 The muscle and tendon fibers of the supraspinatus are positioned anterior to the acromion process, as seen on this axial composite drawing taken from successive MR images. Impingement occurs particularly on the anterior tendon fibers (small arrow) by the anterior inferior acromion (large arrow) when the arm is raised

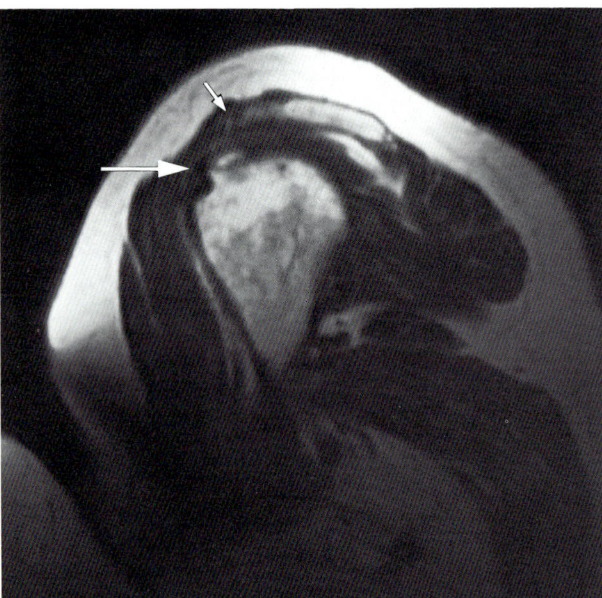

Fig. 4.2 Sagittal T1 image (TR 600/TE 50). Downward spurring of the acromion process (small arrow) and upward spurring of the greater tuberosity (large arrow) severely compromise the space available for the supraspinatus tendon

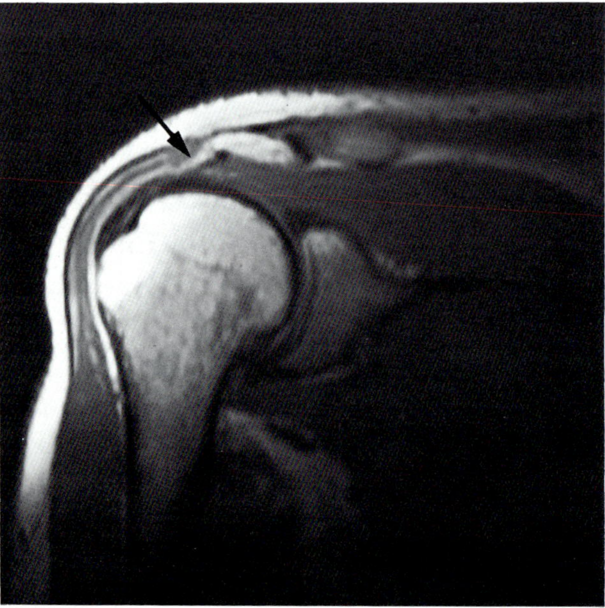

Fig. 4.3 Coronal proton density image (TR 2000/TE 20). There is ample space between the acromion and humeral head except for a thin spur extending downward from the acromion (arrow), impinging on the supraspinatus tendon

overhead motion. Impingement can be suggested on conventional radiographs when spurs project downward from the acromion and/or upward from the humeral head. On MR images, cortical bone appears black rather than white, but spurs can be easily seen if present (Fig. 4.2). It is advantageous in MRI to be able to visualize both the muscle and tendon as well as bone, for a bony spur compressing these will confirm shoulder impingement even if the space for the muscle appears to be adequate otherwise (Fig. 4.3). The space between the acromion and humerus may be narrowed even without spurs, or with only small bony

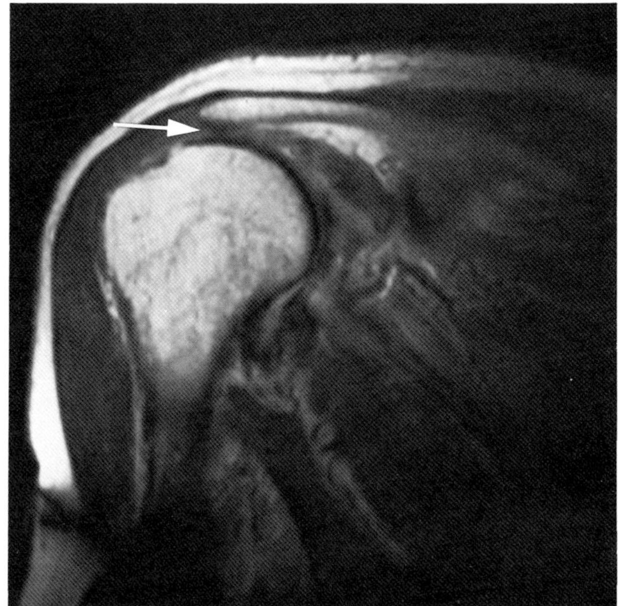

Fig. 4.4 Coronal T2 image (TR 2000/TE 60). The space between the humerus and the acromion is so narrow that even the tiny spur on the latter causes severe impingement (arrow)

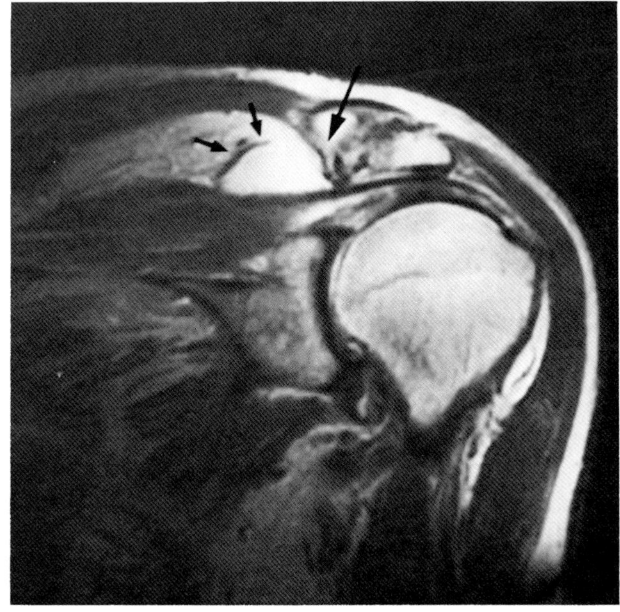

Fig. 4.5 Coronal T2 image (TR 2000/TE 60). Large spur on the inferior acromioclavicular junction markedly depresses the supraspinatus tendon (large arrow). Fluid distends a bursa medial to the spur and above the supraspinatus (small arrows). There is increased signal in the supraspinatus tendon laterally

spurs (Fig. 4.4). Spurring of the acromioclavicular joint may also cause impingement more proximally on the supraspinatus (Fig. 4.5). Pressure on the anterior part of the muscle by the coracoacromial ligament may contribute to shoulder impingement. The ligament is seldom recognized on MR images because it is thin and obliquely oriented to the usual imaging plane. Occasionally it may be demonstrated adjacent to the muscle on sagittal plane images (Fig. 4.6).

The earliest changes made by shoulder impingement on the tendon and muscle are edema and small foci of hemorrhage occurring

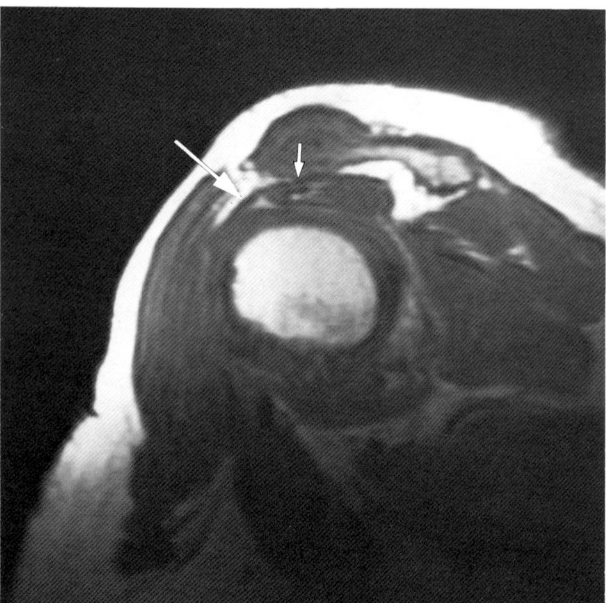

Fig. 4.**6** Sagittal T1 image (TR 800/TE 20). If the coracoacromial ligament (large arrow) is directly adjacent to the supraspinatus muscle (small arrow) as in this patient, it may contribute to shoulder impingement syndrome

in the soft tissue compressed by the overlying bone and ligament. The *compression* affects not only the supraspinatus but the subacromial bursa as well. Swelling of the bursa may contribute to compression of the supraspinatus. This is a grade I impingement syndrome according to the classification developed by Neer (1983; Neer and Welsh, 1977). Since it is the first stage of shoulder impingement, it is seen in younger individuals, often in athletes who use overhead motion of the arm continually such as baseball pitchers, tennis players, and swimmers. Radiographic modalities probably will not demonstrate changes at this stage of

Fig. 4.**7a** Coronal proton-density image (TR 2000/TE 20). Small region of increased signal is present in the lateral supraspinatus tendon (arrow)
b Coronal T2 image (TR 2000/TE 60). Area of abnormal signal becomes much brighter, indicating local edema consistent with tendinitis (arrow)

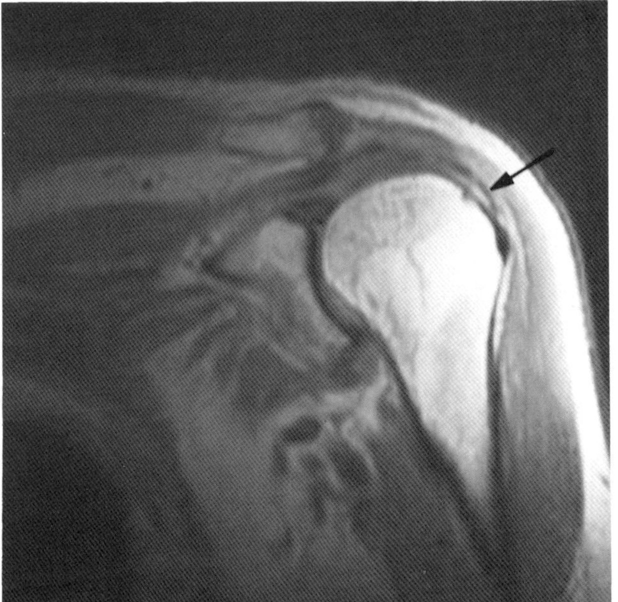

a

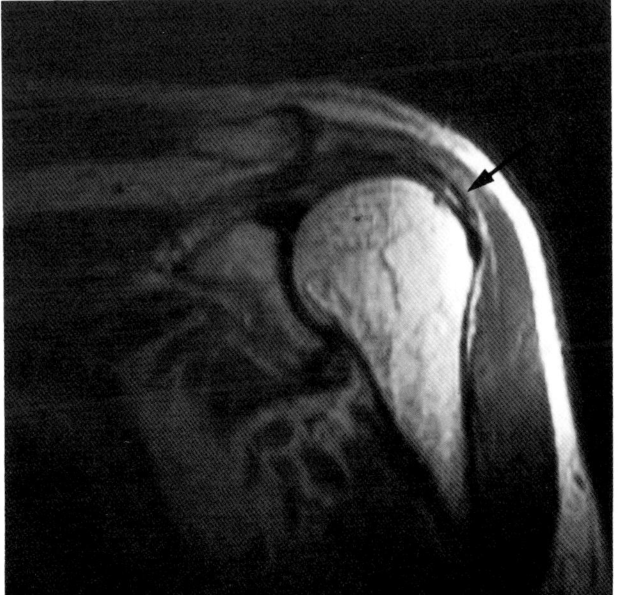

b

shoulder impingement because the acromial spurs or acromioclavicular spurs will not be developed enough to suggest the diagnosis. Shoulder arthrography is of no value at this stage since it outlines only the undersurface of the supraspinatus adjacent to the joint capsule and cannot demonstrate swelling of the tendon or bursa. The diagnosis is based on a positive shoulder impingement test performed by forcing the humerus upward against the acromion and producing pain. Repeating the procedure following subacromial lidocaine injection and producing no pain confirms the diagnosis.

MRI is capable of demonstrating changes in

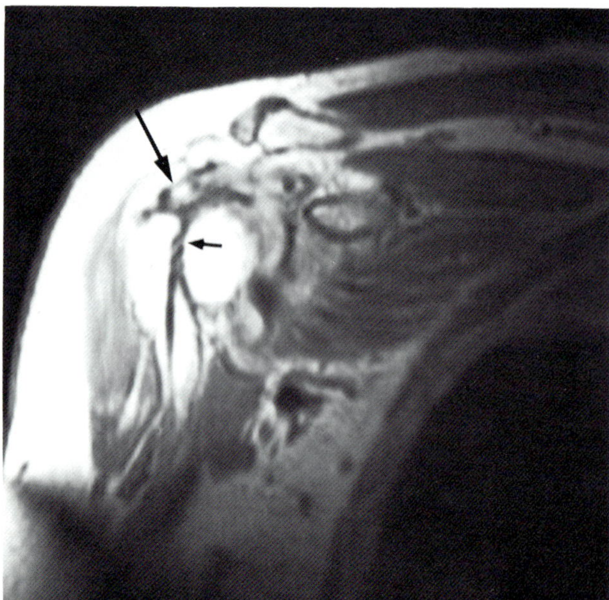

Fig. 4.**8a** Coronal proton-density image (TR 2000/TE 20) and **b** coronal T2 image (TR 2000/TE 60). Small region (large arrow) in anterior supraspinatus tendon which remains bright on both images. Long head of the biceps tendon is seen extending across the humeral head (small arrow)

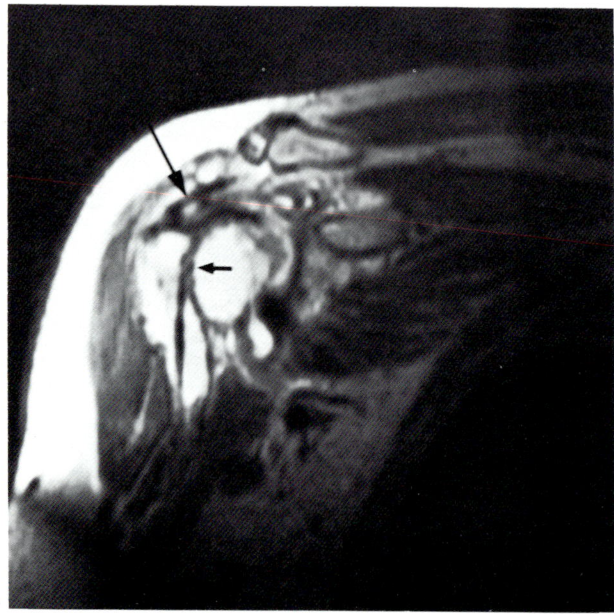

the soft tissue at this stage of impingement. The most subtle finding is a localized region of edema in the lateral supraspinatus muscle fibers or tendon. The edema will have only a slightly lower signal intensity than the muscle fibers if in the muscle, but will appear as a higher signal in the tendon on the images taken with T1 weighting or on short TE–long TR (proton-density) images. Structures with a high water content appear bright on T2-weighted images, and the area of edema will appear considerably whiter than the adjacent muscle and tendon (Fig. 4.**7**). If there is a hematoma with the edema, there will be a region of

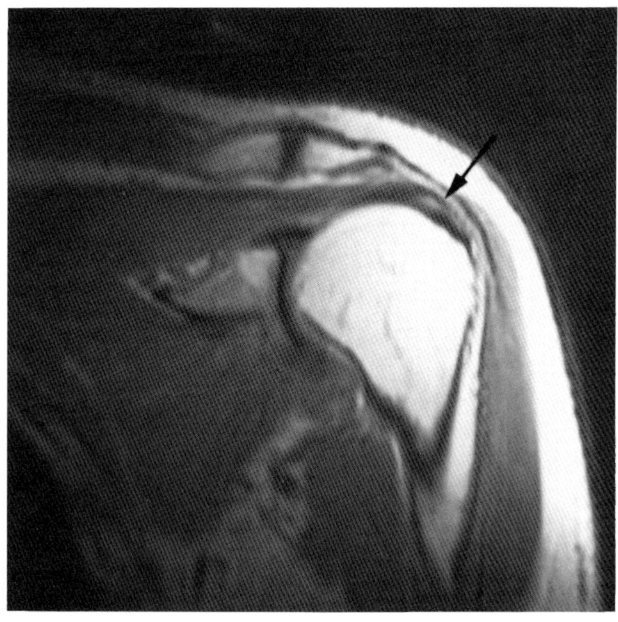

Fig. 4.**9** Coronal proton-density image (TR 2000/TE 20). There is tendinitis with increased signal and swelling in the lateral supraspinatus (arrow)

brightness in the muscle and/or tendon on T1 images which will remain bright on the T2 sequences (Fig. 4.**8**). The muscle or tendon may or may not be swollen at the site of edema and/or hemorrhage (Fig. 4.**9**). The subacromial bursa is not seen under normal circumstances. A thin layer of fat separates the upper border of the supraspinatus from the acromion. If there is swelling with fluid in the subacromial bursa, the signal above the supraspinatus will be the opposite of the usual, namely, low (gray) on the T1 and proton-density images but high (white) on the T2 images because of the fluid (Fig. 4.**10**). This is the opposite of the usual

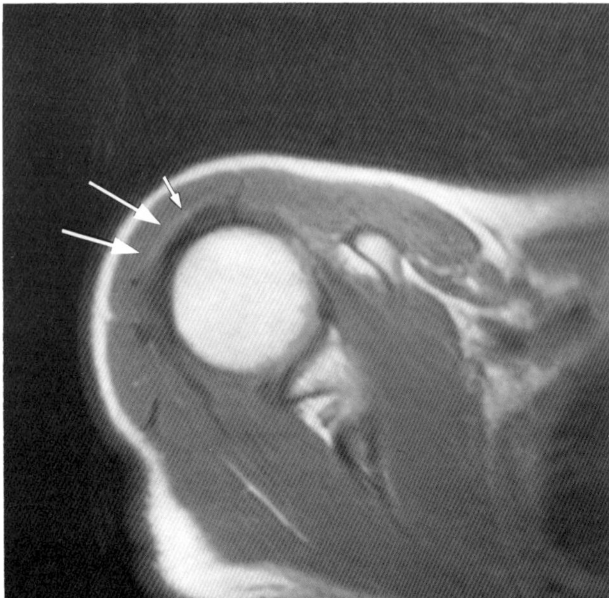

a

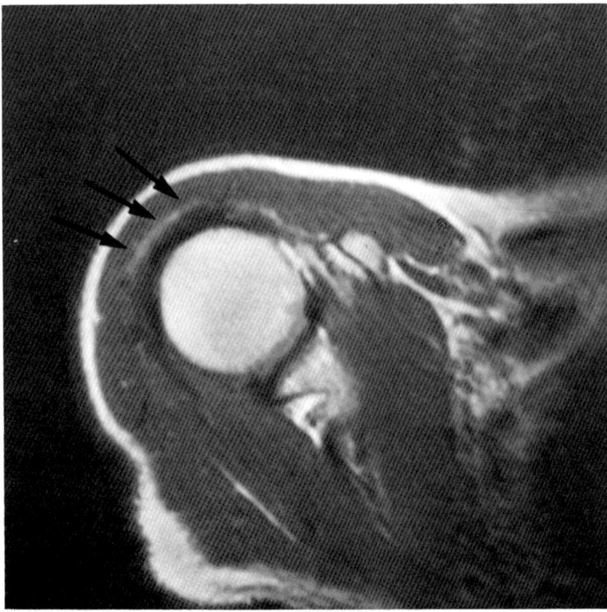

b

Fig. 4.**10 a** Axial proton-density image (TR 2000/TE 20) and **b** axial T2 image (TR 2000/TE 60). The thin rim of fluid indicating bursitis becomes apparent when comparing the bright signal on the T2 image to the same intermediate area of signal on the proton-density image (arrows). The fluid is situated in the subdeltoid bursa, between the deltoid laterally and the supraspinatus attachment to the humerus medially

change of the normal fat in this area from high signal on the T1 and proton-density images to the lower signal on T2 images. If the bursa contains fluid but is not enlarged, this can be a subtle but very helpful finding in the diagnosis.

As the condition of shoulder impingement persists, *fibrosis* and *atrophy* of the muscle/ tendon and the bursa gradually occur. This is grade II of shoulder impingement and obviously will be seen in an older age group than grade I lesions. Fibrotic tissue generally has a low signal intensity on MR images, similar to the normal tendon signal, but there may be variable degrees of persistent edema with early

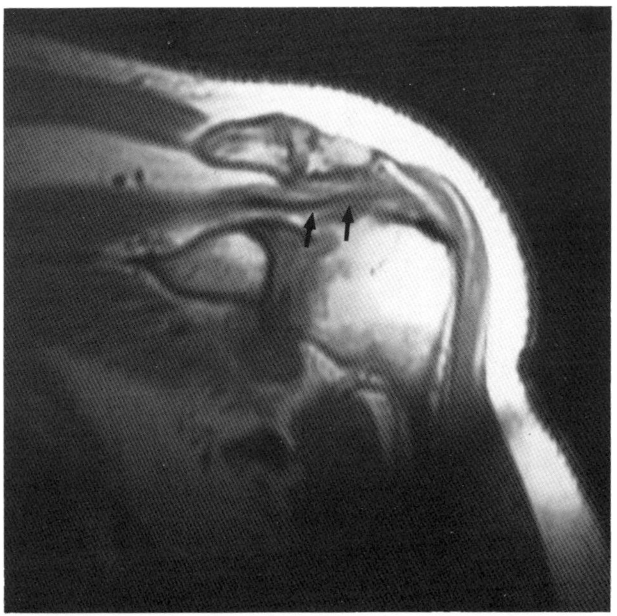

Fig. 4.**11** Coronal proton-density image (TR 2000/TE 20). Narrowing of the supraspinatus tendon with atrophy (arrows). The subacromial bursa above the tendon is of intermediate signal intensity due to fibrosis

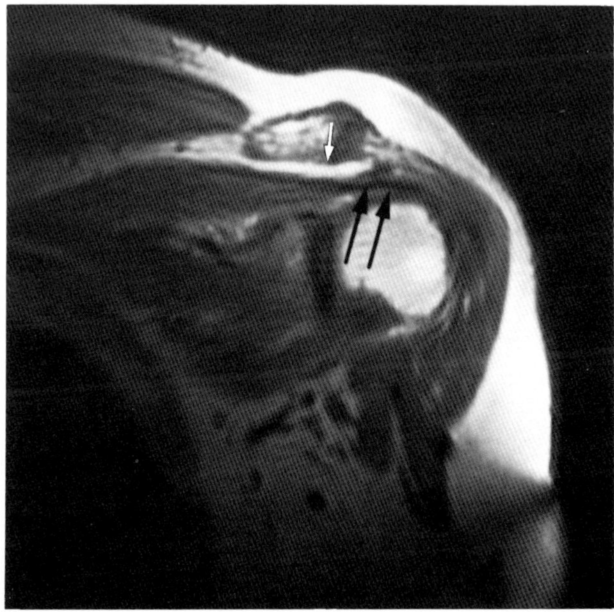

Fig. 4.**12** Coronal proton-density image (TR 2000/TE 20). Narrowed supraspinatus tendon (large arrows). There is fat with high signal intensity in the subacromial bursa region (small arrow)

fibrotic changes, causing the signal to become brighter. The normal fat signal separating the tendon from the acromion may be replaced by lower inhomogeneous signal representing fibrosis in the bursa. As further deterioration occurs, the tendon will become atrophic and narrowed (Fig. 4.**11**). If there is a severe degree of bony shoulder impingement, only the tapered tendon may be visible between the acromion and the humerus. The thickened subacromial bursa may remain visible above the tendon. If the bursa becomes atrophic, the narrowed tendon may be outlined by fat (Fig. 4.**12**). Severe tendon atrophy may be

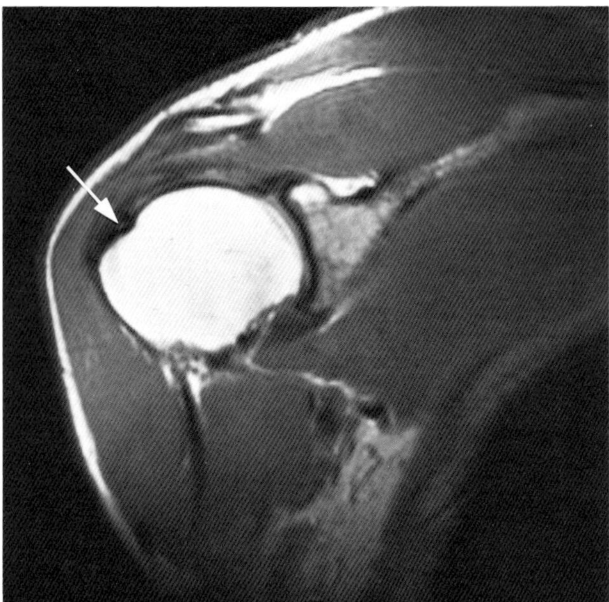

a

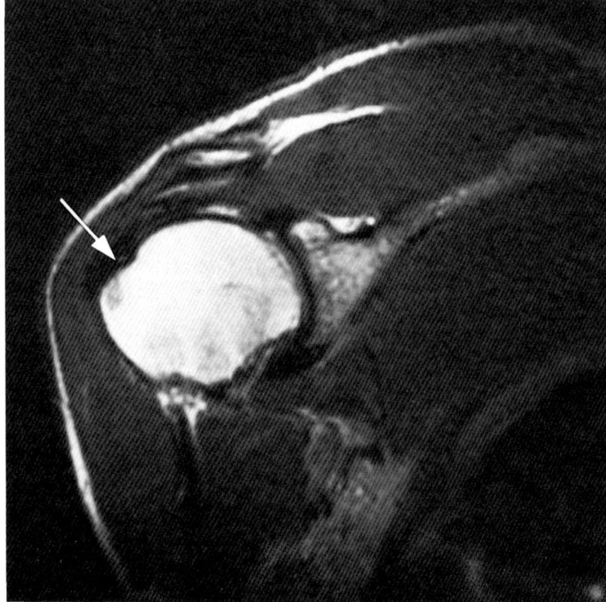

b

Fig. 4.**13a** Coronal proton-density image (TR 2000/TE 20) and
b coronal T2 image (TR 2000/TE 60). A partial tear of the supraspinatus tendon is seen as round intermediate signal intensity on the inferior tendon margin in **a** (arrow). This becomes a bright signal in **b** (arrow)

seen in middle age as an advancing stage of shoulder impingement. In our experience, atrophy without a tear of the tendon is frequently seen in older women.

With continued impingement, the tendon will eventually wear through, producing a *tear* of the rotator cuff. This is grade III of shoulder impingement. An early tear of the cuff may extend only partially through the tendon. The progression from tendinitis to a partial-thickness tear may be experienced as a chronic or gradually increasing pain with abduction of the arm. A sudden increase in pain may herald the disruption of the tendon fibers, but the inciting event may be relatively trivial. Partial tears do not demonstrate an abnormal appearance on

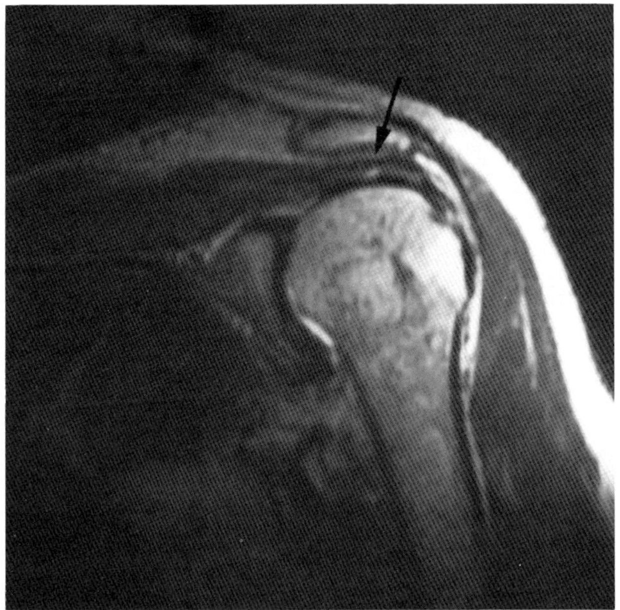

Fig. 4.**14**   Coronal T2 image (TR 2000/TE 60). Bright round signal in the midportion of the supraspinatus tendon consistent with a partial tear (arrow)

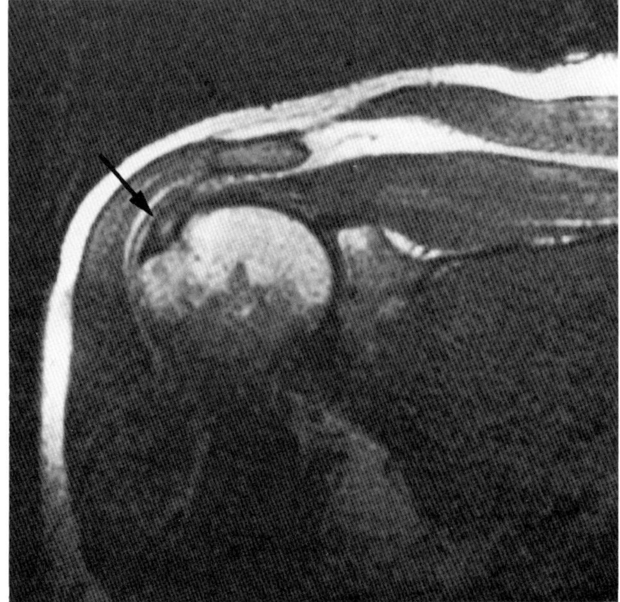

Fig. 4.**15**   Coronal T2 image (TR 2000/TE 60). Moderately bright round signal consistent with a partial tear in the supraspinatus tendon near the insertion on the greater tuberosity (arrow)

an arthrogram unless the tear extends to the inferior surface of the tendon and the irregularity is outlined by contrast. A tear completely confined within the tendon or extending only to the superior surface will not be shown.

Tears of the tendon or muscle are accompanied by edema. Edema has a gray, intermediate signal intensity on T1 and proton-density images; on T2 images, however, it becomes bright and stands out in contrast to the black signal of the tendon or the gray signal of the muscle. Ideally, on an MR image a partial tear will display a linear region of increased signal extending perpendicular or oblique to, and only partially through, the long axis of the tendon fibers. However, a tear may appear as

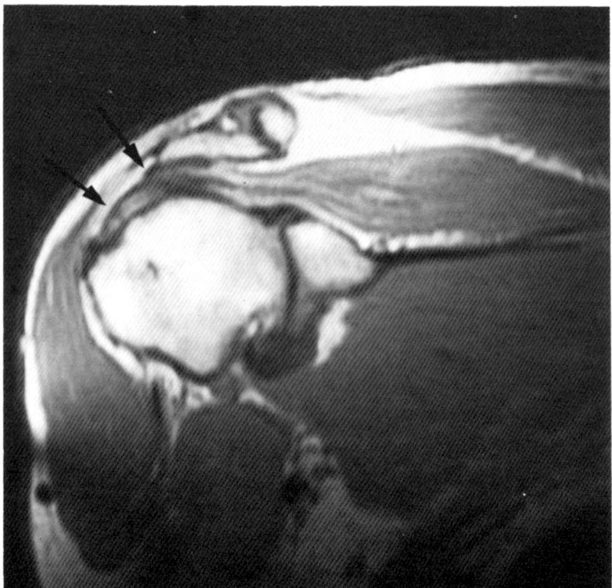

Fig. 4.**16** Coronal proton-density image (TR 2000/TE 20). Intermediate signal within the supraspinatus tendon consistent with a partial tear (large arrow) is present adjacent to an impinging inferior acromial spur (small arrow)

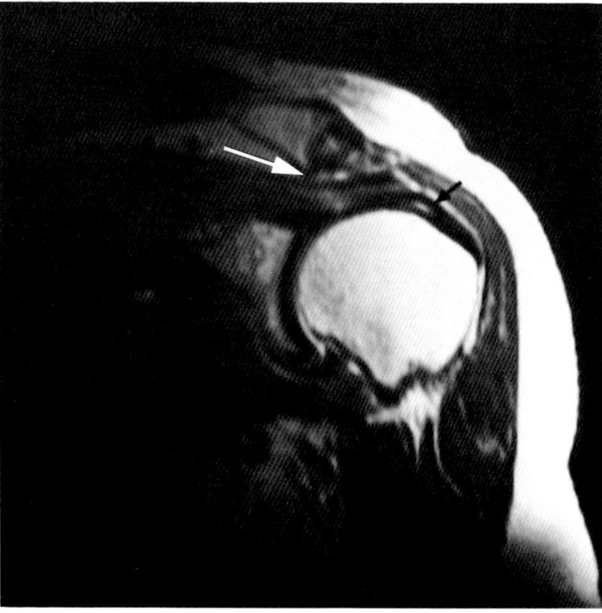

Fig. 4.**17** Coronal T2 image (TR 2000/TE 60). A partial tear of the supraspinatus tendon is present (small arrow). There is also increased signal consistent with inflammatory change in the lateral muscle fibers adjacent to a prominent spur of the acromioclavicular joint (large arrow)

a round area of increased signal extending from the upper or lower margin of the tendon or muscle (Figs. 4.**13–15**). If the tear is juxtaposed to an impinging lesion, such as an acromion or acromioclavicular spur, the diagnosis can be made with more confidence (Fig. 4.**16**). A partial tear of the tendon may be accompanied by inflammatory changes else-where in the tendon or muscle (Fig. 4.**17**). If a partial tear is confined within the tendon and does not extend to the surface, it may be difficult to differentiate from severe tendinitis (Fig. 4.**18**).

The most severe grade III impingement lesion is a full-thickness complete tear through the supraspinatus tendon, which will produce

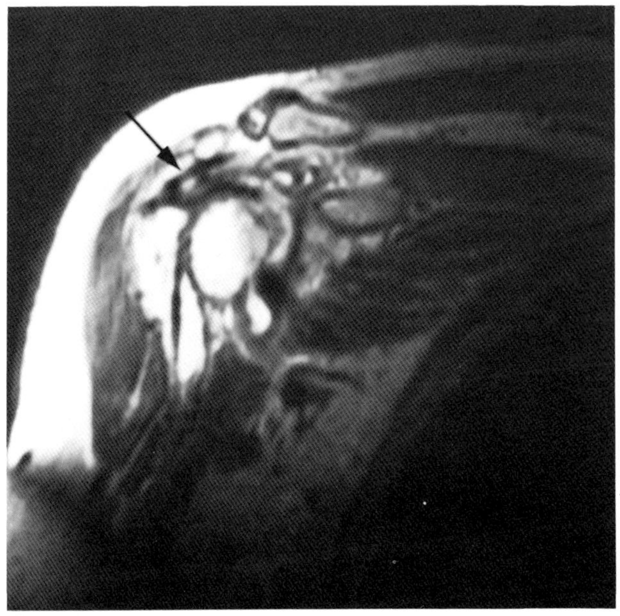

Fig. 4.**18** Coronal T2 image (TR 2000/TE 60). Bright round signal in the anterior fibers of the supraspinatus tendon. This may be due to tendinitis with edema, or may be a partial tear (arrow)

discontinuity of the tendon on the MR image. The joint capsule below and the subacromial bursa above form the fascial boundaries of the supraspinatus. A complete tear disrupts these structures as well, establishing communication between the joint space and the bursa. This condition is the basis for establishing the presence of a rotator cuff tear in shoulder arthrog-raphy. Contrast injected within the joint space will flow into the subacromial and subdeltoid bursae, although the tear itself may or may not be visualized (Fig. 4.**19**). Similarly, a joint effusion can escape into the subacromial and subdeltoid bursae if a full-thickness tear is present. Fluid seen in these bursae is a point in favor of a complete tear, but not definite

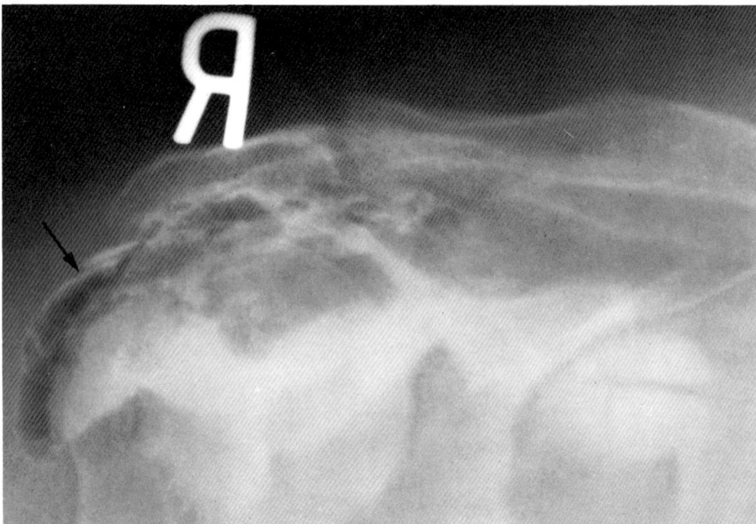

Fig. 4.**19 a** Radiograph of a shoulder arthrogram demonstrating a rotator cuff tear, with air and opaque contrast situated outside of the normal joint space, over the greater tuberosity and lateral humerus (arrow in **a**)
b A normal arthrogram for comparison. The contrast media is confined to the glenohumeral joint space (Courtesy of Dr. Enrique Palacios, Macneal Hospital, Berwyn, Illinois.)

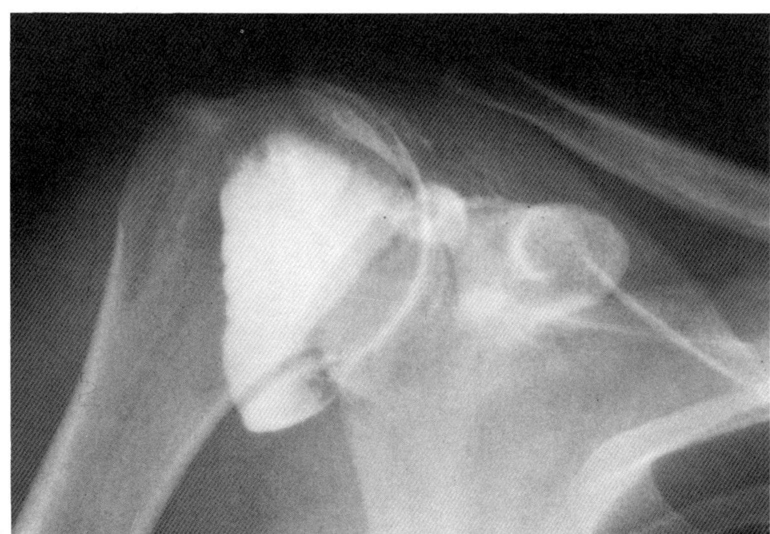

proof, as bursitis would also manifest as fluid in the bursae (Neer and Welsh, 1977).

A full-thickness tear of the supraspinatus that involves only part of the tendon is more common and seen at an earlier age than a total tendon disruption with complete discontinuity. Such a tear may gradually evolve in stages, beginning with a grade I lesion and progressing to grade II (fibrotic, atrophic changes) and partial tears. Indeed, distinguishing a complete tear from a partial tear may not always be possible on an MR scan (Fig. 4.**20**), although the definite establishment of a complete as opposed to a severe partial tear in shoulder impingement may not be of critical importance in management. Complete tears,

Fig. 4.**20** Coronal T2 images (TR 2000/ TE 60). These are the two most anterior images of the coronal series of a 62-year-old man with rotator cuff symptoms. It is unclear whether the abnormal high signal in the supraspinatus tendon is a severe partial tear or if it extends through the full thickness of the tendon (arrows). In arthroscopic examination, a complete tear was found

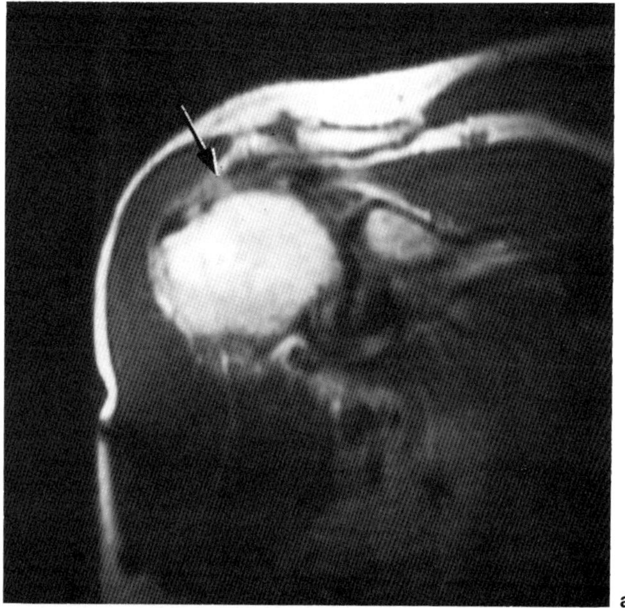

a

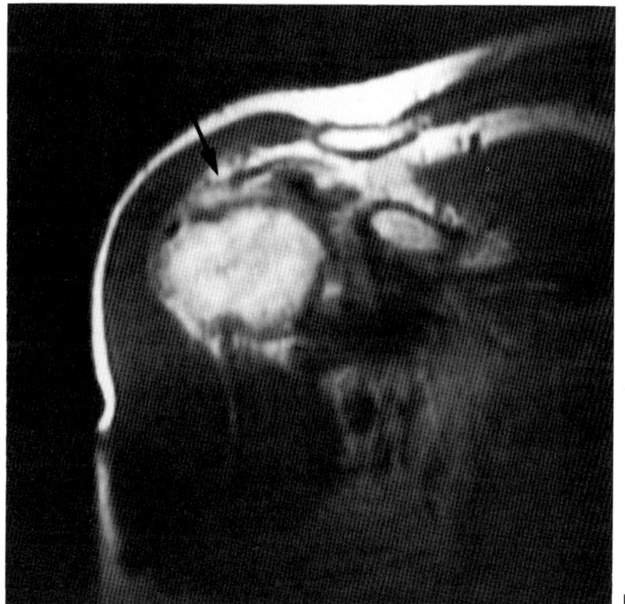

b

like tendinitis and partial tears, tend to occur first in the anterior aspect of the attachment of the tendon to the greater tuberosity. As an early complete tear becomes more severe, involvement of the middle tendon fibers may be seen (Figs. 4.**21**, 4.**22**).

A complete tear may be present in the middle or posterior tendon fibers without involvement of the anterior fibers. If the tear is full thickness but involves only a small section of the tendon, it may be partially seen on several contiguous sections rather than fully seen on a single image (Fig. 4.**23**). In such a case, corroborating evidence such as adjacent impinging spurs or fluid in the subacromial/subdeltoid bursae provide important clues.

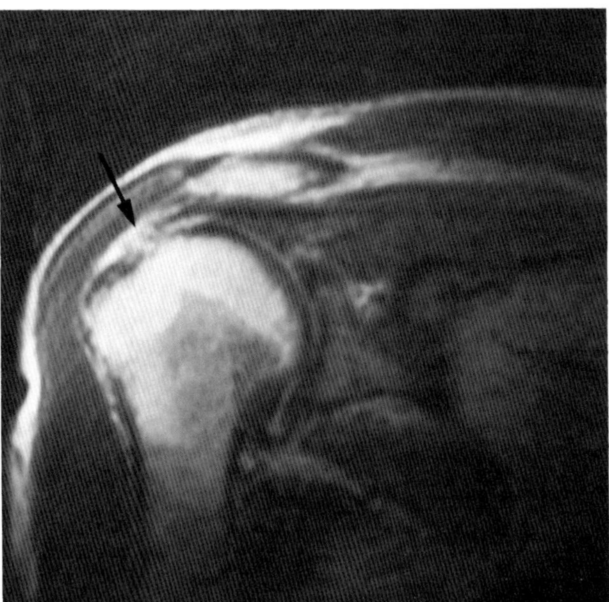

Fig. 4.**21**   Coronal T2 image (TR 2000/TE 60). Full-thickness tear through the middle fibers of the supraspinatus tendon (arrow)

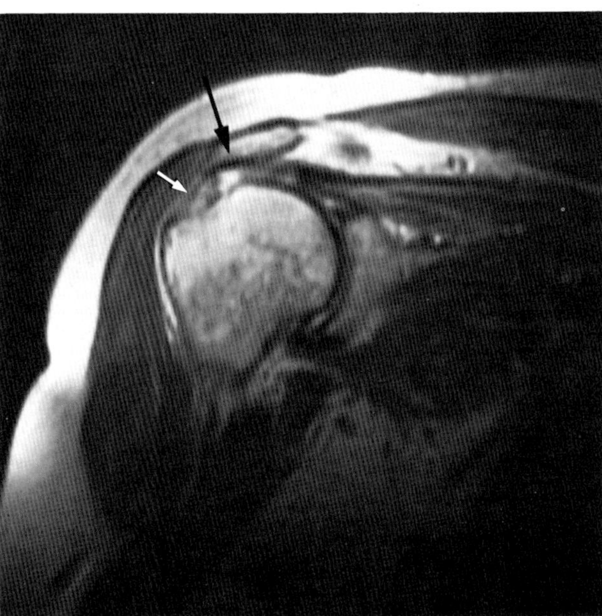

Fig. 4.**22**   Coronal T2 image (TR 2000/TE 60). Full-thickness tear through middle fibers of the supraspinatus tendon (large arrow). Laterally, there is an adjacent region of tendinitis (small arrow)

Fig. 4.**23** Coronal proton density images (TR 2000/TE 20). Full-thickness tear through the supraspinatus is seen extending from the upper aspect of the musculotendinous junction in **a** (arrow) through the midportion (arrows in **b**), and to the inferior surface of the muscle (arrow in **c**). The images are contiguous sections; **c** is the furthest posterior

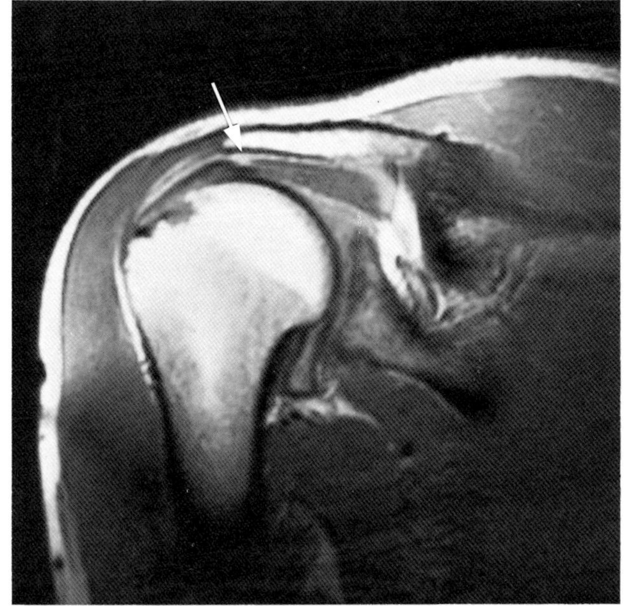

a

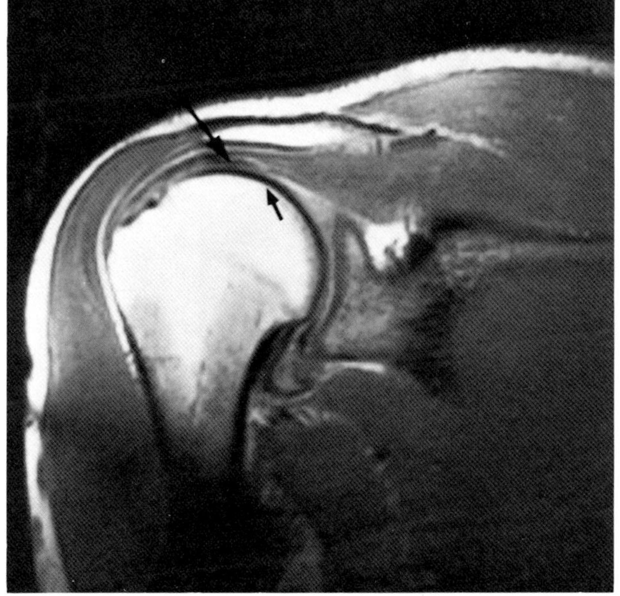

b

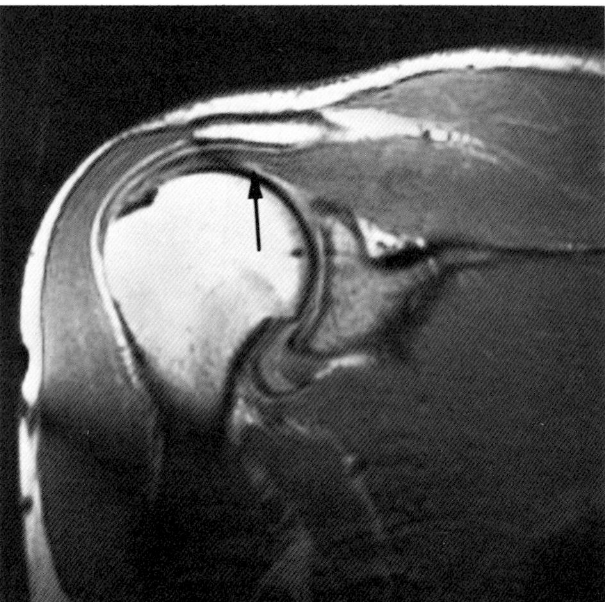

Fig. 4.**23 c**

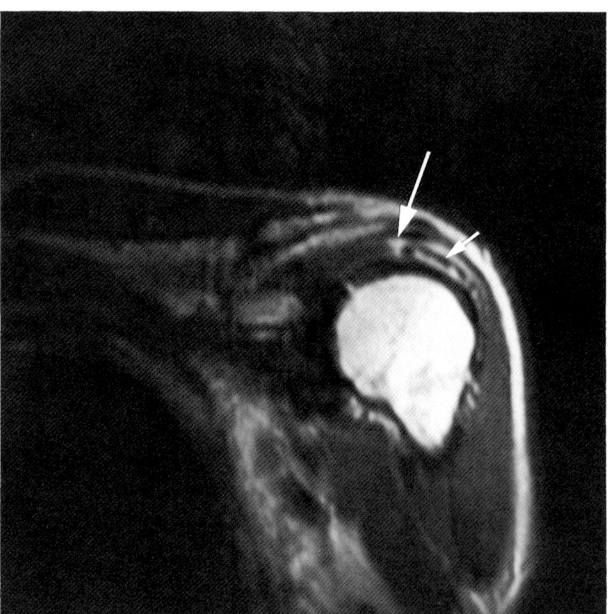

Fig. 4.**24** Coronal T2 image (TR 2000/ TE 60). Complete tear through the supraspinatus musculotendinous junction (large arrow) is associated with high signal intensity edema of the tendon lateral to the tear (small arrow)

A complete tear in one part of the tendon may be associated with the earlier changes of edema or fibrosis in another part of the tendon (Fig. 4.**24**). Degenerative sclerotic or cystic changes in the greater tuberosity may accompany the rotator cuff tear (Figs. 4.**25**, 4.**26**).

With complete disruption of the supraspinatus tendon there is free communication between the joint space and the subacromial/ subdeltoid bursae. Unless traumatic in origin, a total tear of the muscle is usually seen in upper middle-aged to elderly persons. Bony changes of shoulder impingement are often evident (Fig. 4.**27**). Without the attachment to the greater tuberosity, the muscle will tend to contract toward its origin on the supraspinatus

Fig. 4.25 Coronal T2 image (TR 2000/TE 60). Sclerotic degenerative area in the anterior greater tuberosity is seen as a low-signal region on the MR scan (large arrow). Adjacent bright signal is fluid in the subdeltoid bursa in a patient with a complete rotator cuff tear (small arrow)

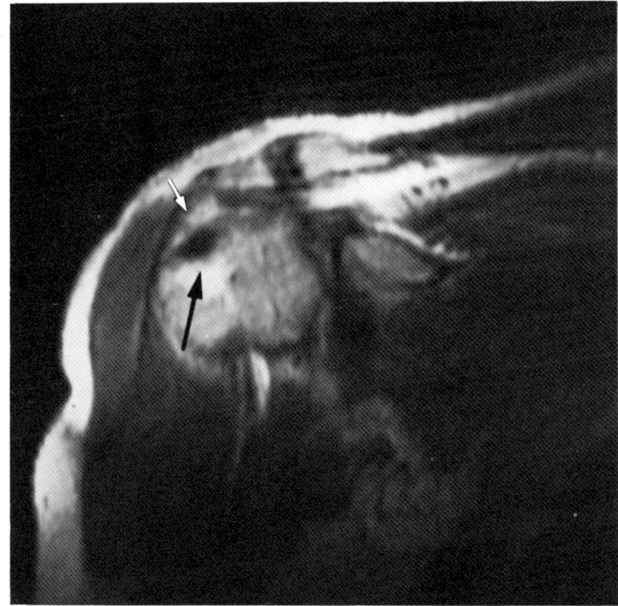

Fig. 4.26 Coronal T2 image (TR 2000/TE 60). Cystic degenerative change in the greater tuberosity (large arrow) adjacent to a full-thickness tear of the supraspinatus tendon (small arrow)

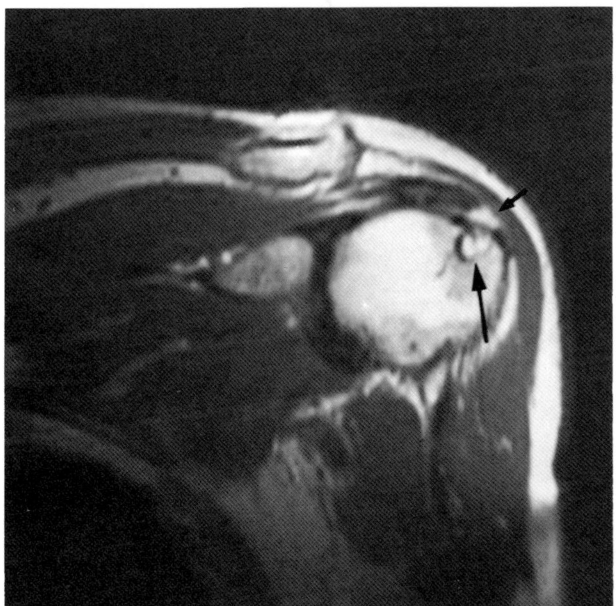

fossa of the scapula (Fig. 4.**28**). The longer the condition prevails, the more atrophic the supraspinatus will become, further widening the distance between the torn muscle border and the humerus, making surgical repair increasingly difficult (Fig. 4.**29**). In long-standing cases, the retracted fibrotic supraspinatus may be difficult to identify, and the large rotator cuff tear will be evident on axial-plane as well as coronal-plane sections. Chronic effusion in the subdeltoid bursa is not infrequently seen (Fig. 4.**30**). Effusions may also be present in other bursae around the shoulder (Figs. 4.**31**, 4.**32**).

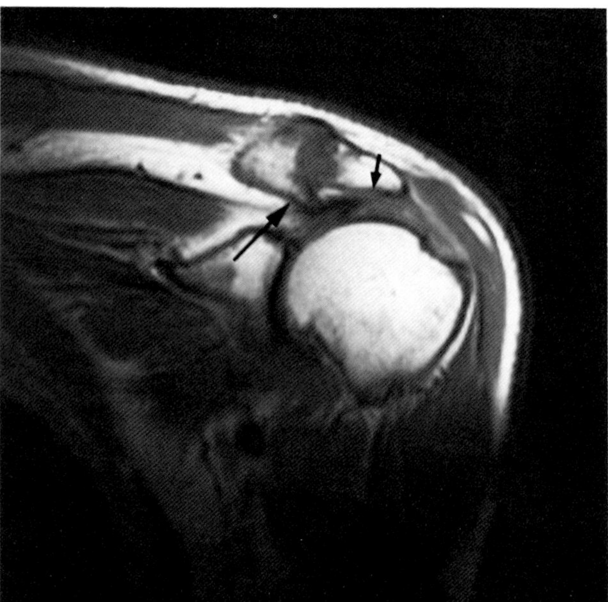

Fig. 4.**27**   Coronal proton-density image (TR 2000/TE 20). Prominent inferior spur on the lateral clavicle (large arrow) is accompanied by detachment of the tendon from the greater tuberosity (small arrow)

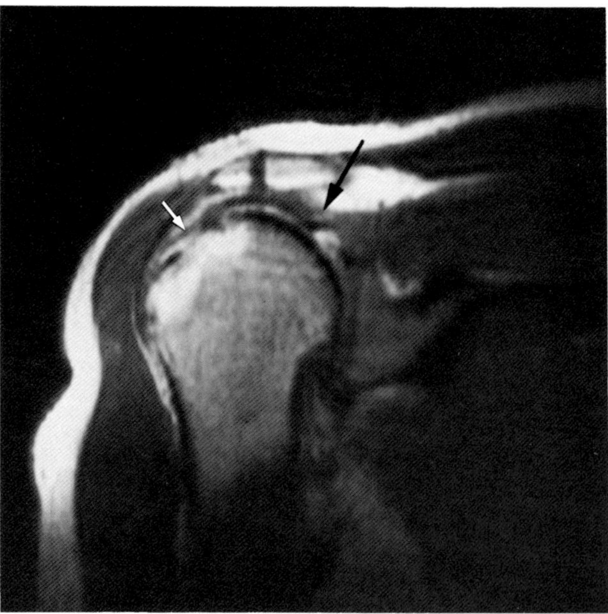

Fig. 4.**28**   Coronal T2 image (TR 2000/TE 60). Lateral muscle fibers of the supraspinatus are atrophic and retracted (large arrow). The tendon is also atrophic (small arrow), and further anteriorally there is a full-thickness tear

Fig. 4.**29**   Coronal T2 image (TR 2000/TE 60). Supraspinatus (arrows) is atrophic and retracted toward its origin in the supraspinatus fossa with a long-standing complete tear of the rotator cuff

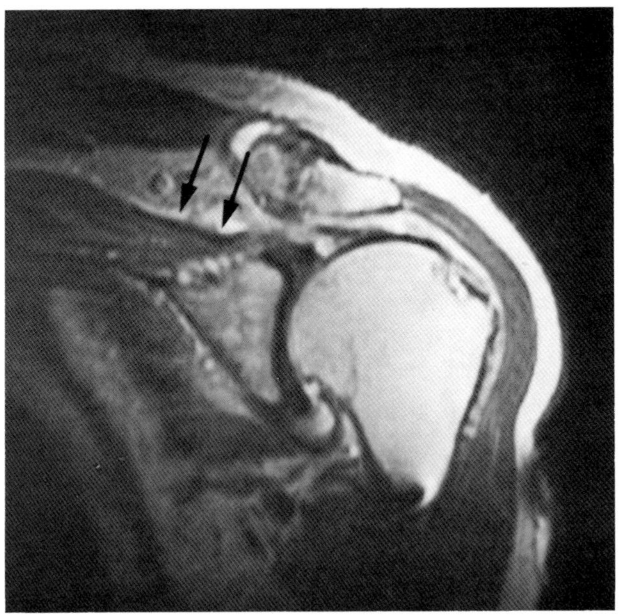

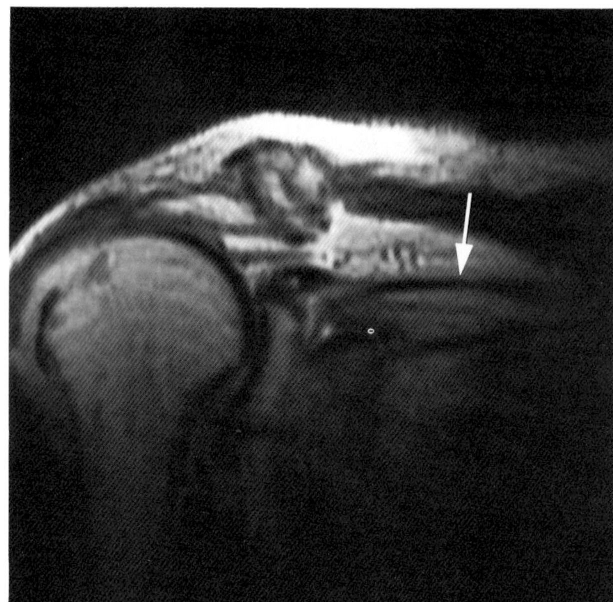

a

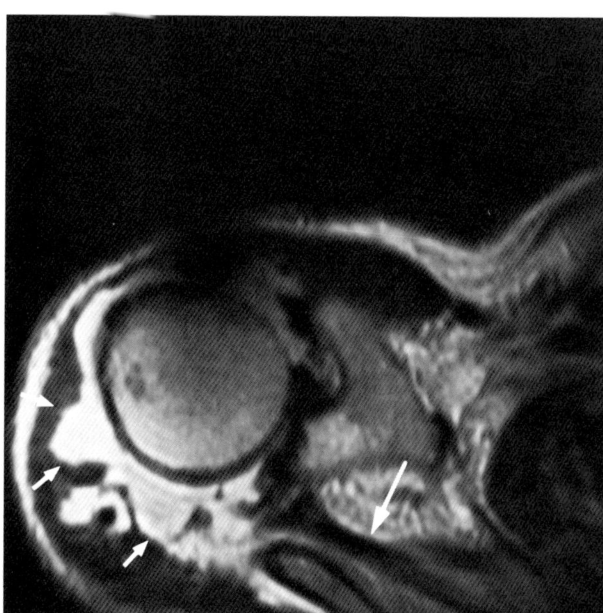

b

Fig. 4.**30 a**   Coronal T2 image (TR 2000/TE 60). Long-standing complete tear of the rotator cuff in an 86-year-old man. The muscle has mixed low and moderately high signal, representing fibrotic strands with interspersed edematous muscle fiber (arrow)

b   Axial T2 image (TR 2000/TE 60). Same patient as in **a**. The thin fibrotic remnant of the supraspinatus is seen with higher-signal edematous muscle fibers more medially (large arrow). There is a large subdeltoid bursa effusion with a scalloped appearance (small arrows)

Fig. 4.**31a** Coronal proton-density image (TR 2000/TE 20) and **b** coronal T2 image (TR 2000/TE 60). Fluid is present in a bursa under the atrophic and torn supraspinatus tendon. The fluid can be distinguished from fat and muscle because it has a gray intermediate signal on the proton-density image (arrows in **a**), which becomes a high white signal on the T2 image (arrows in **b**)

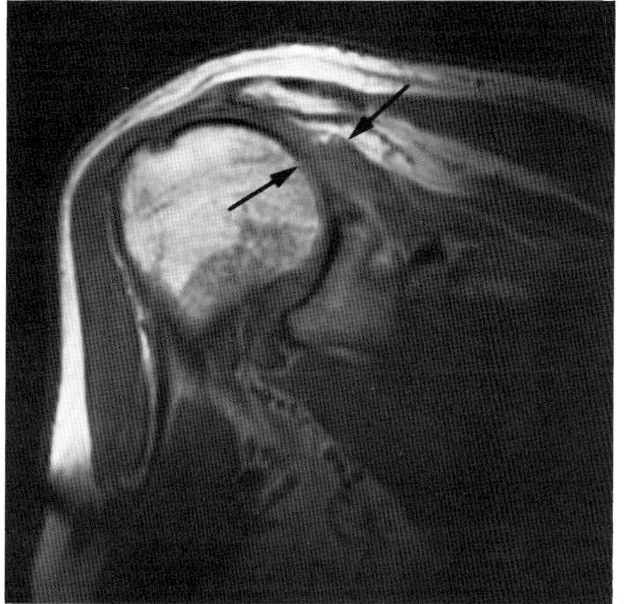

a

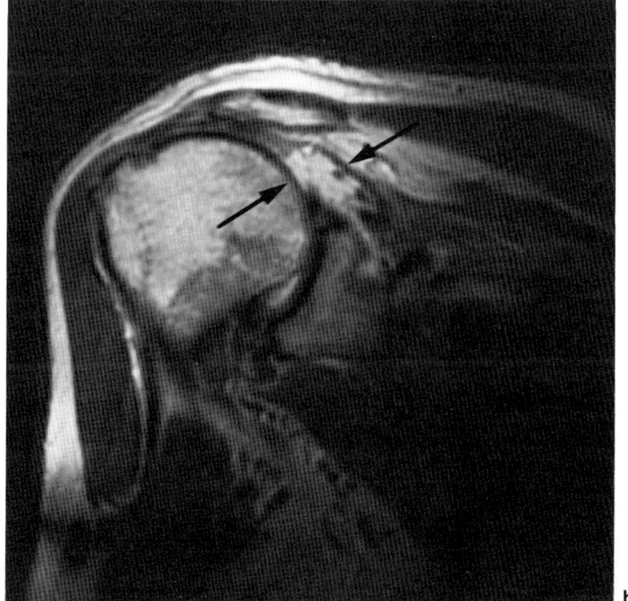

b

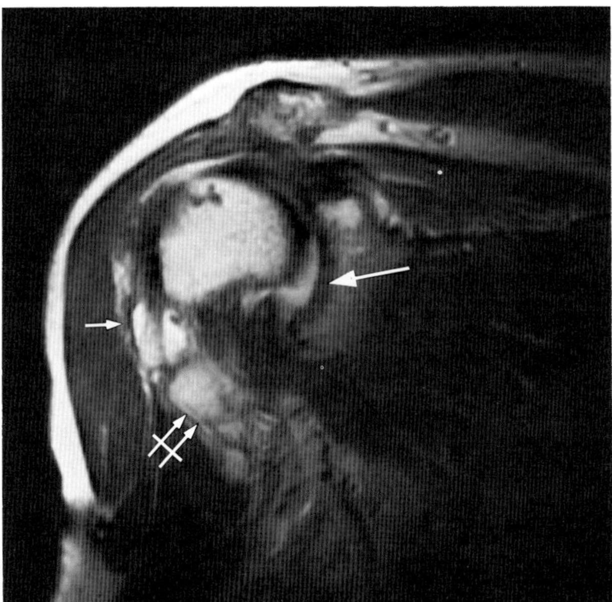

a

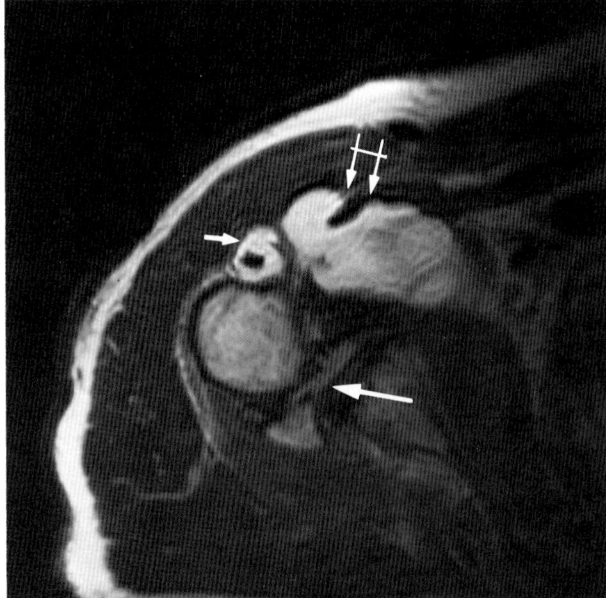

b

Fig. 4.**32a**   Coronal T2 image (TR 2000/ TE 60). Fluid is present in the joint space (large arrow), in the sheath of the long head of the biceps tendon (small arrow), and in a bursa anterior to the subscapularis muscle (double arrow) in a patient who has a full-thickness supraspinatus tear
b   Axial T2 image (TR 2000/TE 60). Same patient as in **a**, showing fluid in the joint space (large arrow), in the sheath of the long head of the biceps tendon (small arrow), and in a bursa anterior to the subscapularis muscle (double arrow)

One cause of rotator cuff tears is shoulder impingement with subsequent degenerative changes of the tendons. This is most often observed in persons over 45; a high incidence is associated with advancing age. However, a tear can occur acutely through injury, which is more frequently seen in younger individuals. Any or all of the tendons of the rotator cuff may be involved, and there is usually a definite history of trauma. A fracture of the greater tuberosity of the humerus is probably a more common cause than soft-tissue injury alone. An avulsion fracture of the greater tuberosity will be accompanied by a tear of at least a portion of the rotator cuff (Fig. 4.**33**).

The infraspinatus muscle attaches to the

Fig. 4.**33** Coronal proton-density image (TR 2000/TE 20). Detached tendon of the supraspinatus is present adjacent to an irregular indentation of the greater tuberosity (arrow), suggesting that a previous avulsion fracture caused the detachment. The patient is a 39-year-old man who did not recall a specific injury

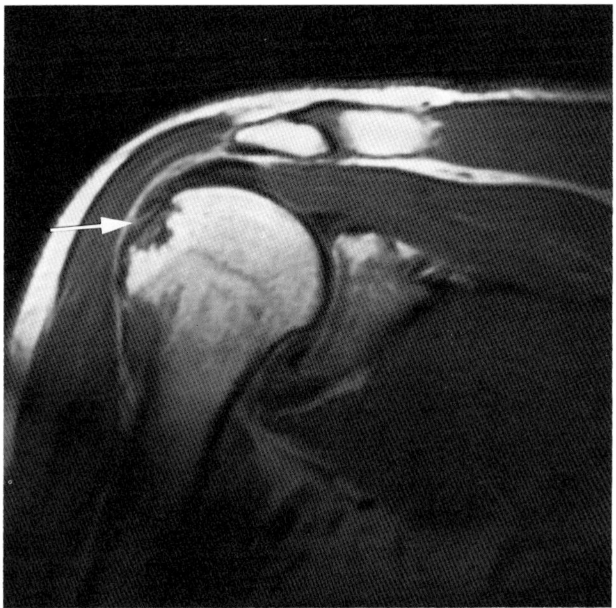

Fig. 4.**34** Axial T2 image (TR 2000/TE 60). There is swelling and a partial tear of the lateral fibers of the infraspinatus (arrows) in a patient who had a complete disruption of the supraspinatus attachment

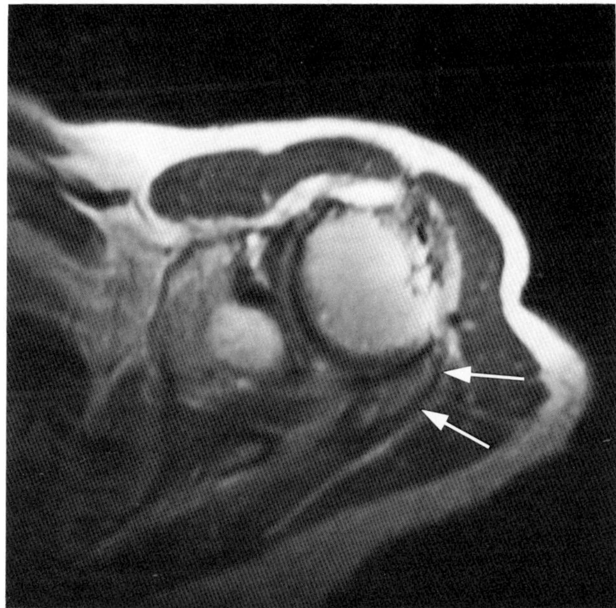

greater tuberosity on its middle facet, just below the attachment of the supraspinatus. A large supraspinatus tear can extend into the tendon of the infraspinatus; this would be demonstrated by an increased signal in the tendon on the T2 images and by discontinuity (Fig. 4.**34**). A rotator cuff tear involving only the infraspinatus is unusual, and trauma rather than shoulder impingement syndrome would be a more likely cause. If the rotator cuff tear is severe enough, extension through the teres minor tendon, which inserts on the lowest facet of the greater tuberosity, may also be present, though rarely. Chronic tears through these muscles may result in atrophy and muscle retraction toward their origins on the

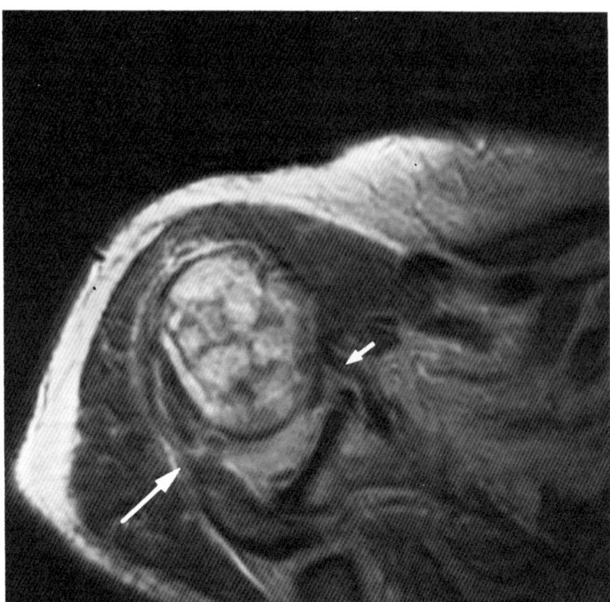

Fig. 4.**35**   Axial T2 image (TR 2000/TE 60). This patient was a 58-year-old man previously involved in an automobile accident. The subscapularis tendon is atrophic and partially detached from the lesser tuberosity (small arrow). The infraspinatus is torn (large arrow). Numerous irregular low-signal lines through the medullary cavity of the humeral head are due to trabecular bone fractures. There is a large joint effusion

scapula. With severe trauma, most probable after sudden shoulder dislocation, a rare complete disruption of all four tendons of the rotator cuff can occur. Not surprisingly, this appearance may be accompanied by fractures of the humeral head or glenoid (Fig. 4.**35**).

The tendon of the long head of the biceps muscle attaches to the superior rim of the glenoid on its bony surface, and also on the adjacent fibrocartilaginous rim of the glenoid labrum. It forms a curve along the anterosuperior humeral head, and then extends inferiorly within the bicipital groove. An extension of the joint capsule accompanies the tendon down the groove to the junction with the muscle fibers. The upper portion of the

Fig. 4.**36a** Axial T2 image (TR 2000/TE 60). Fluid distends the capsular extension of the long head of the biceps tendon (arrow). No joint effusion is present
b Coronal T2 image (TR 2000/TE 60). High-signal fluid in the sheath surrounds the long head of the biceps tendon as it courses over the humeral head (arrow)

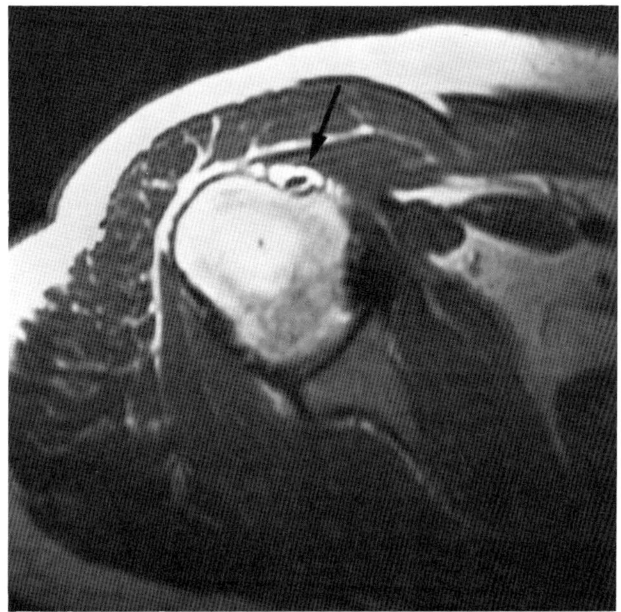

a

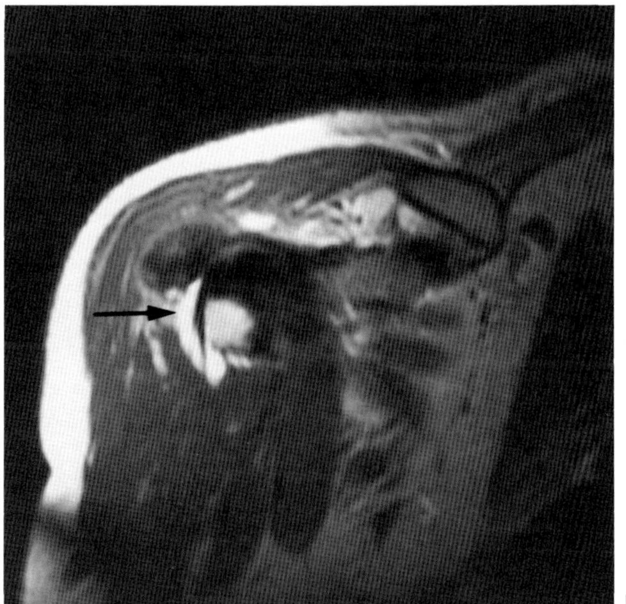

b

tendon extending along the upper humeral head is within the joint capsule and may be subjected to the same stresses from degenerative changes and shoulder impingement as the supraspinatus tendon, which lies in close proximity above it. This can lead to bicipital tendinitis, causing pain anteriorly over the shoulder. This condition may be difficult to dif- ferentiate clinically from, and may indeed coexist with, rotator cuff degenerative changes. This may result in thinning of the tendon within the bicipital groove, and be accompanied by an effusion within the adjacent capsular extension forming the tendon sheath (Fig. 4.**36**). Eventually, a complete tear of the long head of the biceps tendon may occur, usu-

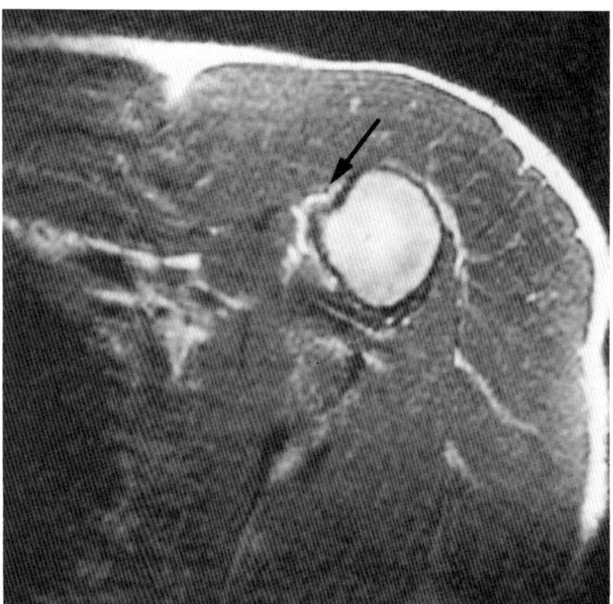

a

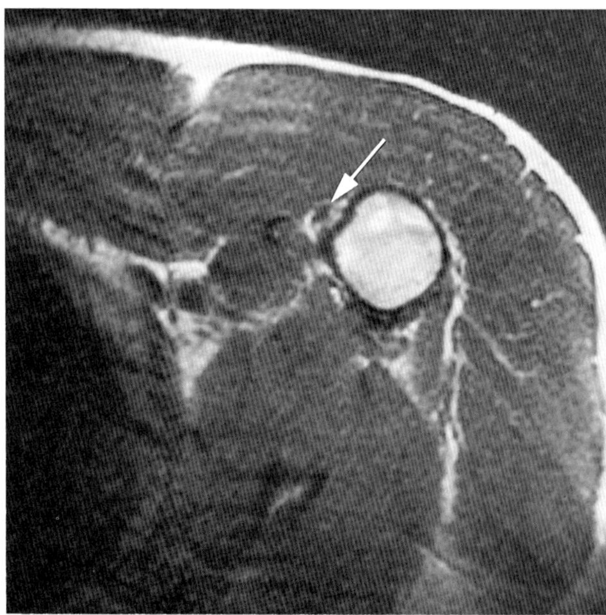

b

Fig. 4.**37** Axial T2 images (TR 2000/TE 60). The patient is a 44-year-old man with the clinical findings of a rupture of the long head of the biceps tendon. In **a** the tendon appears diminished but not absent (arrow) suggesting a partial tear. The next image, taken inferiorly (**b**), shows the normal size and appearance of the tendon below the site of the tear (arrow)

ally in the act of forceful flexion of the elbow. This allows the long head of the biceps to contract distally forming a round prominence under the skin of the upper arm when the elbow is flexed. In MRI, the tendon sheath in the bicipital groove may be easily seen, especially on T2 images, because of distention with fluid. The black dot normally seen representing the proximal tendon sheath will be absent along the upper humerus, but will appear on more distal sections (Fig. 4.**37**).

The tendon of the long head of the biceps is normally held in check in the bicipital groove by a covering of fibrous tissue, a fascial extension of the tendons of the subscapularis and pectoralis major muscles, and by the trans-

Fig. 4.**38** Axial proton-density image (TR 2000/TE 20). There is medial dislocation of the long head of the biceps tendon (arrow). There is a very shallow bicipital tendon groove of the humerus which predisposes the patient to this condition

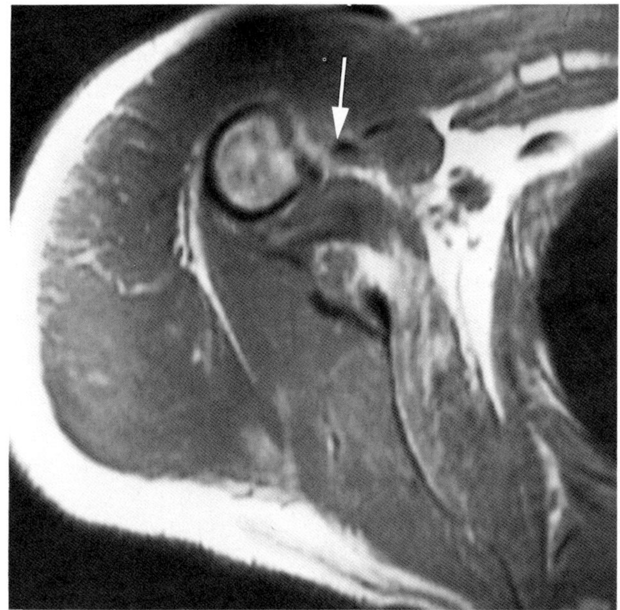

Fig. 4.**39** Axial proton-density image (TR 2000/TE 20). The long head of the biceps tendon is absent from its normal position along the anterior humerus, but instead is seen medially (arrow)

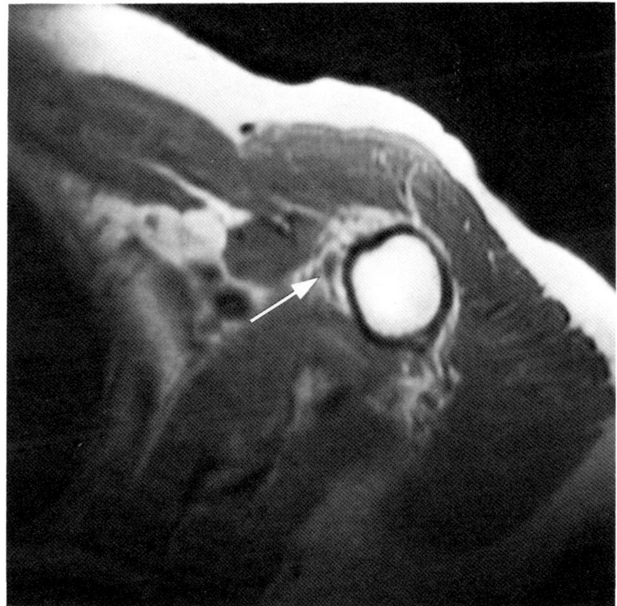

verse humeral ligament extending between the greater and lesser tuberosities. If degenerative changes cause disruption of the fibrous covering, dislocation of the tendon may occur. Since its proximal attachment is to the glenoid, the dislocation will always occur medially. This is most commonly seen in middle-aged or older individuals. A shallow bicipital tendon groove predisposes one to the condition (Fig. 4.**38**). The dislocation may occur with external rotation of the arm. Reduction of the tendon back into the bicipital groove spontaneously with internal rotation may or may not occur. If reduction does occur, there may be an audible and painful snap as the tendon slides across the medial ridge of the bicipital groove. If the dis-

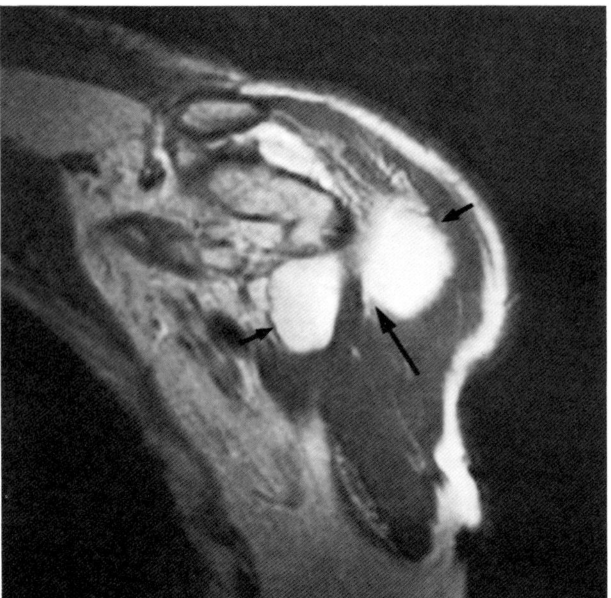

Fig. 4.**40**   Coronal T2 image (TR 2000/TE 60). The long head of the biceps tendon is medially displaced from the tendon groove (large arrow), and extends directly downward from its origin on the superior glenoid rim. There is fluid in the tendon sheath (small arrows)

located tendon does not reduce, the bicipital groove will be empty, as in the case of tendon rupture, but the tendon may be seen in a more medial position along the anteromedial surface of the humerus. This is best observed on the axial-plane image (Fig. 4.**39**), but may also be seen on the modified coronal views (Fig. 4.**40**).

Degenerative changes and vascular compromise to the rotator cuff may lead to dystrophic calcium deposition in the tendons of the rotator cuff, again most frequently in the supraspinatus. A painful inflammation of the involved tendons may ensue, particularly with rapid calcium accumulation. With acutely inflamed calcium deposits, pain will be present

Fig. 4.**41 a**   Coronal proton-density image (TR 2000/TE 20). Prominent low signal of the supraspinatus tendon is due to calcific tendinitis (arrow)
b   Radiograph of the same patient, which demonstrates the calcification of the supraspinatus tendon (arrow)

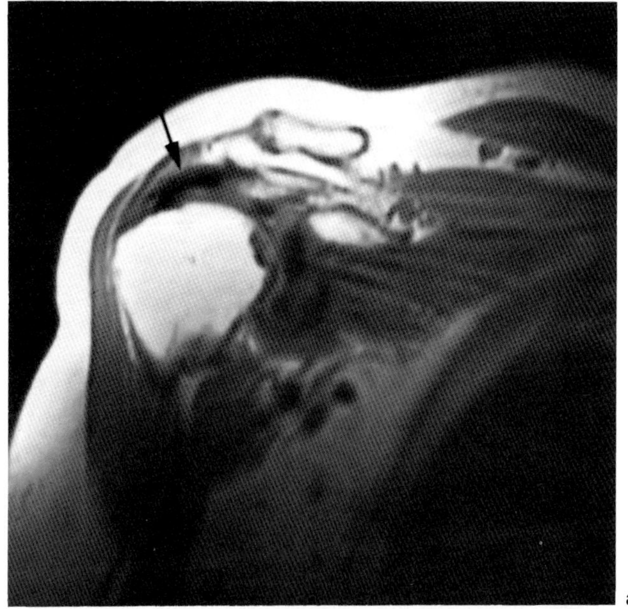

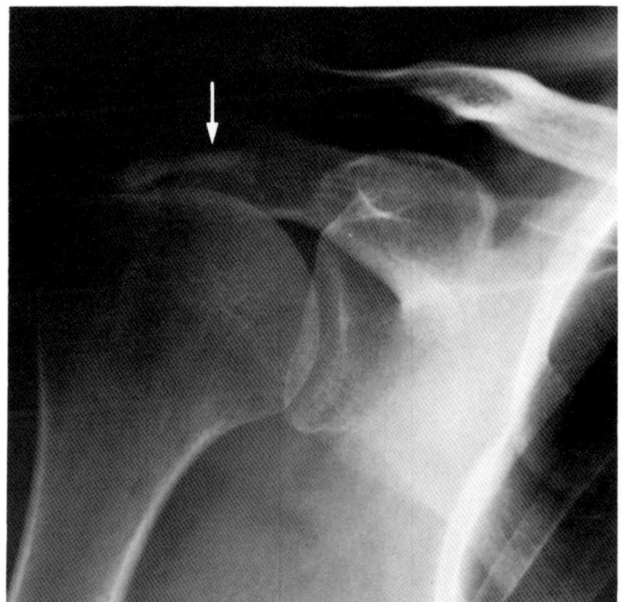

at rest, but exacerbated by any movement of the shoulder. The overlying bursae may become secondarily inflamed and swollen, worsening the condition with further shoulder impingement. The acute process may resolve when the amorphous calcium salt deposits in the tendon extrude into the bursae, where they will become reabsorbed. Calcific tendinitis may occur more gradually as well, with less severe pain but more chronicity.

Calcium deposits appear dark on MR scans, and may be impossible to differentiate from the normal low signal of the tendon. If the deposit widens or causes irregularity of the margin of the tendon, then it can be detected. (Figs. 4.**41**, 4.**42**). If an acute inflammatory

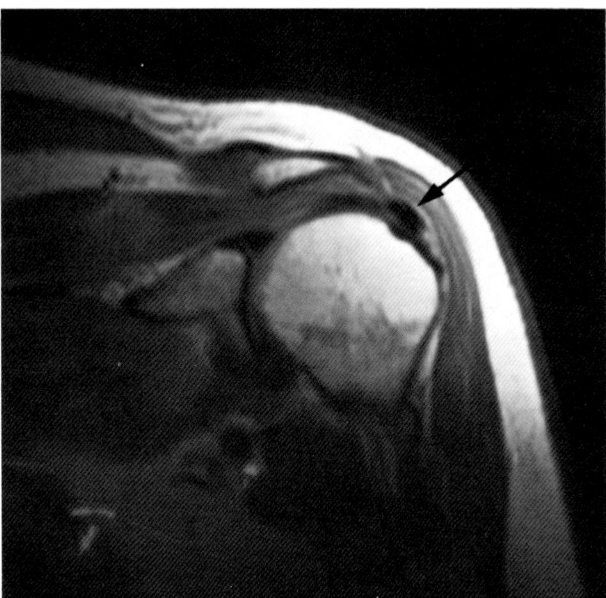

Fig. 4.**42a** Coronal proton-density image (TR 2000/TE 20). Calcific tendinitis of the supraspinatus, with calcified deposits partially protruding into the subdeltoid bursa (arrow)
b Axial proton-density image (TR 2000/TE 20). Same patient as in **a**, with a localized region of calcific tendinitis of the supraspinatus (arrow)

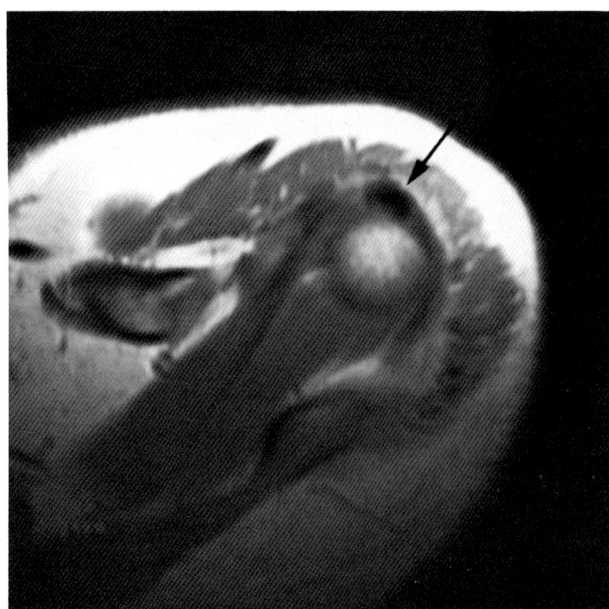

process is present, there may be fluid or edema of the subacromial bursa, with high signal intensity. Amorphous calcium deposits may occur elsewhere in soft tissues other than the tendons, in regions of prior trauma or inflammation, or for unknown reasons (Fig. 4.**43**).

Dislocation, subluxation, and *instability* are common problems of the shoulder. The shoulder is the most mobile joint in the human body, but consequently the most unstable joint as well. The glenoid fossa is shallow and there is only a small area of the humeral head in contact with the glenoid at any position of the arm. The fibrocartilaginous labrum circumferentially surrounds the rim of the bony glenoid to provide a bit more depth to the fossa. The

Fig. 4.**43 a** Radiograph demonstrating a round calcified density adjacent to the coracoid process in a 46-year-old woman who complains of shoulder pain with no known history of trauma or infection at this site
b Coronal T2 image (TR 2000/TE 60). Amorphous calcific deposit contains areas of intermediate signal with central dark regions, suggesting that it is partially of fibrous tissue (arrow). A portion of the clavicle is above the lesion and the coracoid process below

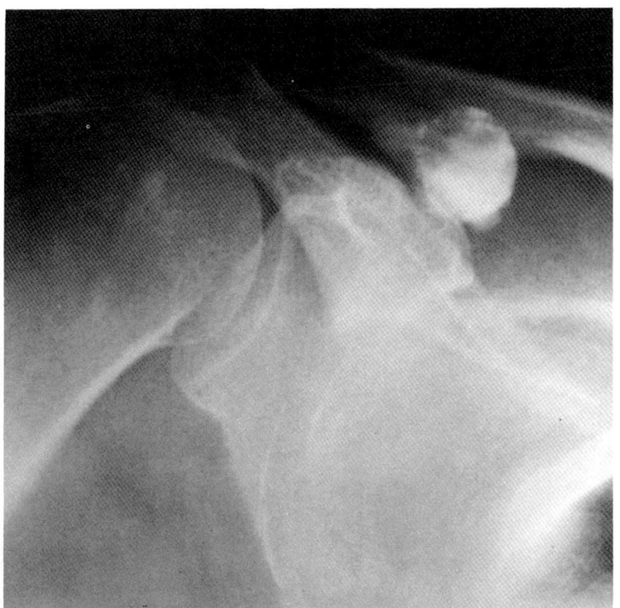

a

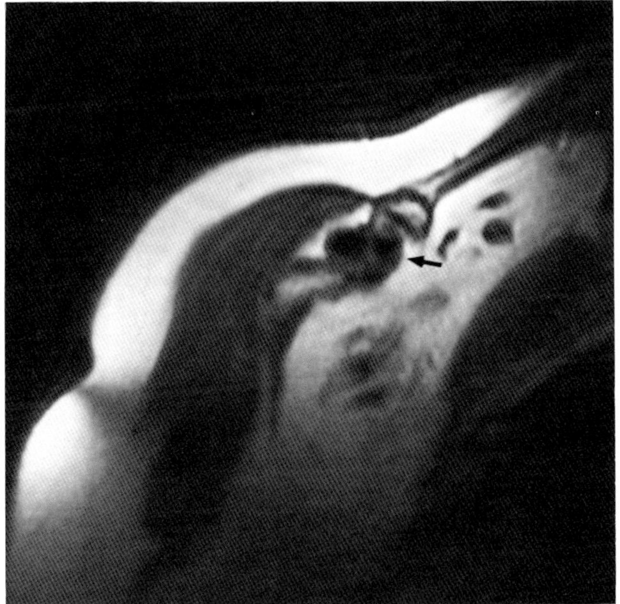

b

integrity of the joint is dependent on the surrounding soft-tissue structures. The joint capsule itself is rather thin, strengthened by the glenohumeral ligaments which are fibrous thickenings of the capsule itself. There are usually three ligaments situated in a superior, middle, and inferior arrangement. The muscles of the rotator cuff surround the anterior, superior, and posterior sides of the joint, blending with the capsule and further reinforcing its stability. The tendon of the long head of the biceps may aid in this process as well. Finally, several strong ligaments are present external to the rotator cuff. The coracoacromial ligament may aid joint stability, though, as mentioned previously, it may cause shoulder

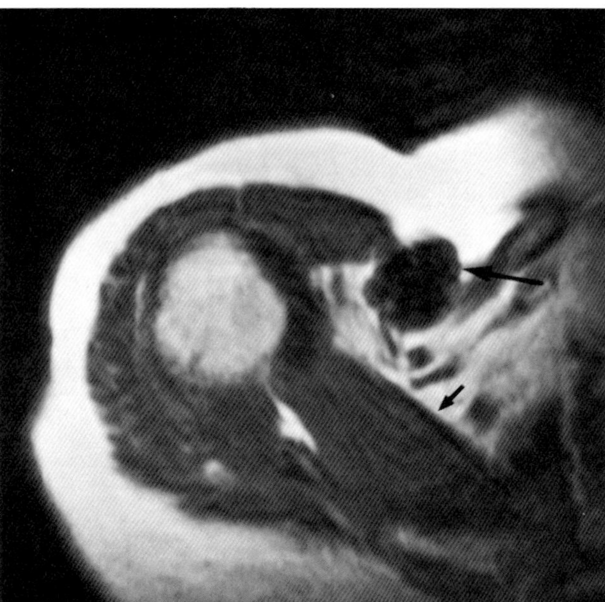

Fig. 4.**43c**   Axial T2 image (TR 2000/TE 60). The round calcified deposit (large arrow) is anterior to the supraspinatus (small arrow)

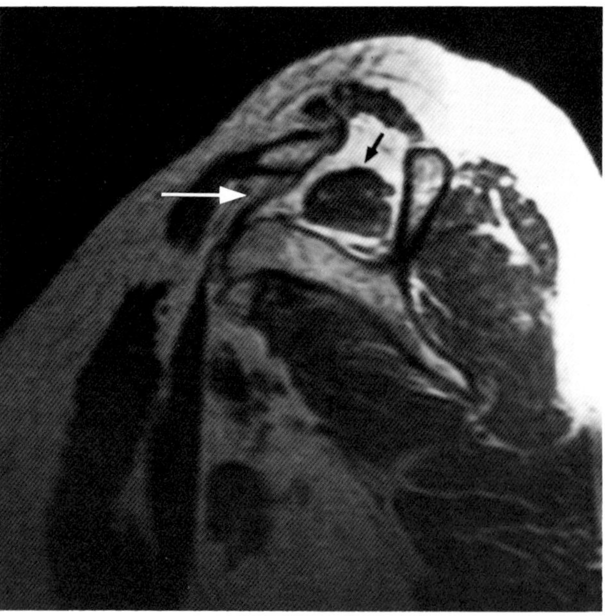

Fig. 4.**44**   Sagittal T1 image (TR 800/TE 20). The coracoclavicular ligament (large arrow) and its relationship to the supraspinatus muscle (small arrow) is well demonstrated

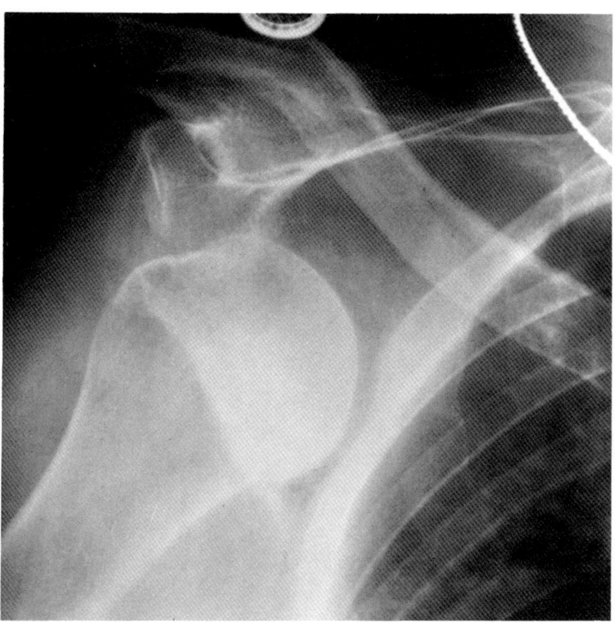

Fig. 4.**45**   Radiograph of an anterior dislocation of the humerus. The humeral head is projected over the inferior glenoid and under the coracoid process

impingement and worsen rotator cuff degenerative symptoms. The coracoclavicular ligament is a strong band divided into trapezoid and conoid sections (Fig. 4.**44**, see also Fig. 2.**3**). This contributes to joint stability by preventing upward subluxation of the clavicle. MRI evaluation adds a dimension that has not previously been available for the assessment of these problems.

The most frequent direction of displacement of the shoulder is anteriorly. This occurs when there is forward stress on an arm which is in abduction and hyperextension. This usually occurs in young, active individuals. A sudden sharp pain at the moment of dislocation is felt, followed by limited mobility with inability to adduct the arm. Conventional radiographs will show the dislocated humeral head obviously not in contact with the glenoid fossa, often lying under the coracoid process. In the process of dislocation, the humeral head will forcibly cross the margin of the glenoid. This may cause a tear of the cartilaginous portion of the labrum, or may even cause a fracture of a portion of the bony rim attached to the labrum. A fractured anterior rim of the glenoid and/or glenoidal labrum constitutes the Bankart deformity. As the humeral head dislocates an-

teriorly, it is driven downward by the adjacent coracoid process, but the surrounding muscles and ligaments of the shoulder prevent further downward excursion. As a result, the humeral head will be forced against the anterior aspect of the glenoid. If the pressure of the impingement is sufficient, an impacted fracture of the humeral head will result, characteristically in its posterior superior aspect, which is known as the Hill–Sachs deformity.

The joint capsule attaches medially to the glenoidal labrum. In young individuals with anterior dislocation, a capsular tear will likely occur at this attachment. Healing of the tear may not occur with reduction of the dislocation (Reeves, 1968). If healing does spontaneously occur, the capsule may reattach at a more medial location along the scapula rather than at the labrum. The result is a lax joint capsule anteriorly which predisposes to recurring instability and dislocation. The position of the anterior attachment of the capsule to the scapula is sometimes given a grading system, with grade I indicating a normal attachment to the rim, and grades II and III representing progressively more medially attaching joint capsules.

The subscapularis tendon also lends stability

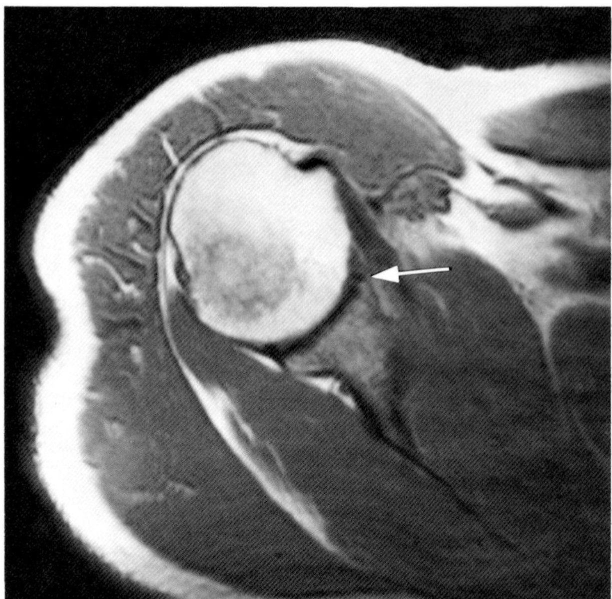

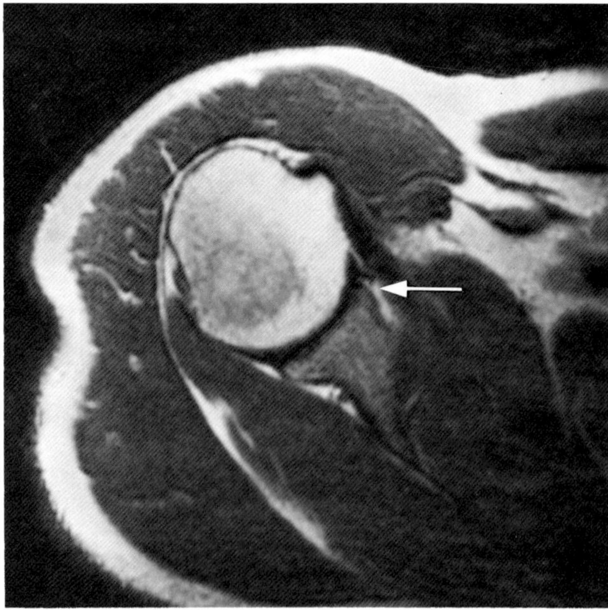

Fig. 4.**46a** Axial proton-density image (TR 2000/TE 20), and **b** axial T2 image (TR 2000/TE 60). A small tear of the anterior cartilage of the labrum is present and separated from the attached cartilaginous rim by an intermediate signal in **a** (arrow), which becomes high signal and is better appreciated in **b** (arrow)

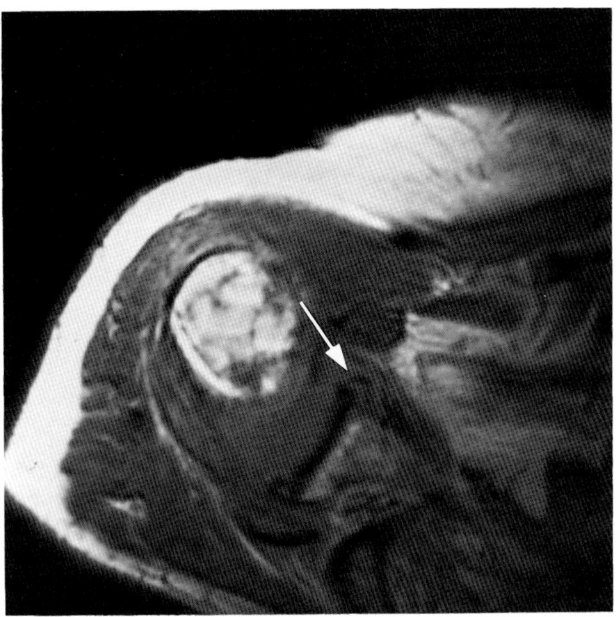

Fig. 4.**47** Axial proton-density image (TR 2000/TE 20). A fragment of the torn glenoid lies slightly separated from the rim of cartilage in the anterior joint space (arrow)

to the shoulder joint anteriorly (Symeonides, 1972). Anterior dislocation can lead to stretching or tearing of the tendon, which may then remain lax following spontaneous healing and allow continued anterior instability. The subscapularis bursa deep to the tendon normally communicates with the joint space through an opening between the glenohumeral ligaments. Postdislocation subscapularis laxity allows the bursa to widen, particularly if there is a joint effusion, thus furthering continued instability.

If a radiograph is obtained during an episode of anterior dislocation, there is usually little problem in establishing the diagnosis since the humerus is displaced below and medial to the glenoid fossa (Fig. 4.**45**). Following reduction, the shoulder may appear completely normal, or a Hill–Sachs deformity of the humerus may be present. If the dislocation has caused a fracture of the rim of the bony glenoidal labrum, this should be visible on conventional radiographs but is in practice often difficult to distinguish from the underlying bone unless the fracture line is directed perpendicular to the plane of the radiograph. Similarly, a tear of the fibrous labrum may eventually result in dystrophic calcification of the fragment, a sign occasionally seen with a

history of previous dislocation or an unstable shoulder. The calcification may also be hard to recognize on conventional shoulder films unless it is not projected on the underlying bone.

Because of the precipitating trauma and extreme pain suffered by the patient during a traumatic dislocation, MRI is not likely to be the initial modality of evaluation. A patient with a prior history of dislocation is usually referred for MRI because of continued pain, a subjective feeling of instability with fear of subluxation, or recurrent dislocation. With MRI, any residual damage caused by the dislocation can be assessed, and this evaluation may contribute to the decision on whether to treat surgically or conservatively.

The anterior margin of the glenoidal labrum is a frequent site of damage after anterior dislocation. Normally the glenoid is examined best on axial MR images and can be seen as a triangular structure of low signal intensity extending from the bony margins of the glenoid fossa (see Fig. 2.**6d**). A tear of the fibrocartilage will appear as an area of intermediate signal intensity on the proton-density images and of high signal intensity on the T2 images (Fig. 4.**46**). The outline of the cartilage may otherwise be intact. In more severe disruption,

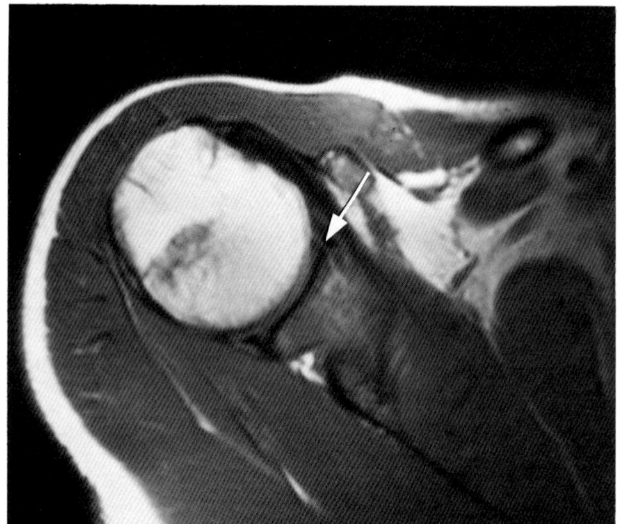

Fig. 4.**48 a** Axial proton-density image (TR 2000/TE 20) and **b** axial T2 image (TR 2000/TE 60). A thin rim of hyaline cartilage of intermediate signal intensity (arrows) which separates the darker fibrocartilage of the glenoidal labrum from the bone is seen on both the proton-density and T2 images

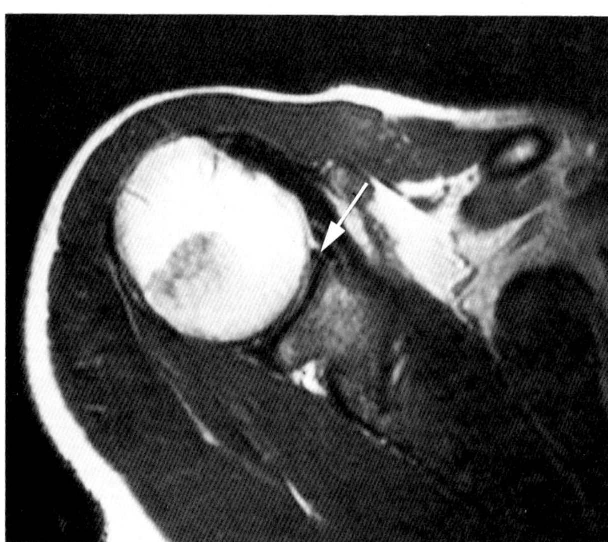

a fragment of the cartilage may separate from the main portion and lie either partially or totally free in the joint space (Fig. 4.**47**). The hyaline cartilage of the glenoid fossa underlying the labrum may sometimes be seen as a prominent line of increased signal separating the labrum from the bone and should not be mistaken for a torn labrum (Fig. 4.**48**). Failure to visualize the labrum in the superior aspect

of the joint does not necessarily indicate a deformity from dislocation. The labrum may be small or absent around the superior rim of the glenoid fossa (Fig. 4.**49**).

If the force producing the dislocation is severe enough, the bony rim of the glenoid may be fractured along with the labrum. Even if healing occurs, a blunted, deformed anterior glenoid can be recognized (Fig. 4.**50**). The op-

Fig. 4.**49** Axial proton-density image (TR 2000/TE 20). There is absence of the fibrocartilaginous rim of the labrum anteriorly near the upper aspect of the glenoid

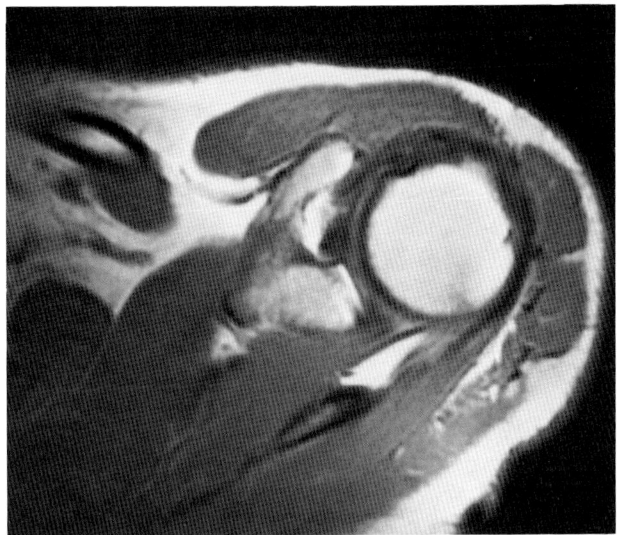

Fig. 4.**50** Axial proton-density image (TR 2000/TE 20). Deformity of the anterior bony margin of the glenoid is present (arrow). The patient is a 36-year-old man with a history of anterior dislocation 19 years previously, with subsequent anterior instability

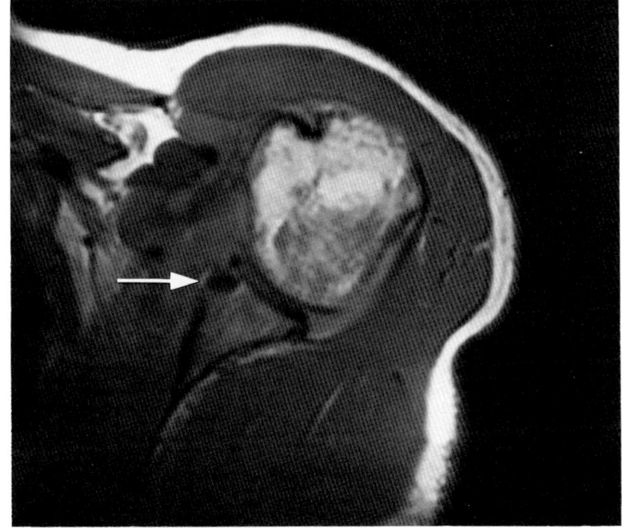

posite appearance, a hypertrophied glenoidal labrum with overgrowth and spurring, is sometimes seen as the result of a less severe degree of anterior instability (Fig. 4.**51**).

If the anteriorly dislocated humeral head is compressed against the rim of the glenoid, a compression cortical fracture, or Hill–Sachs defect, may occur on the lateral and upper aspect of the humeral head. This is best seen on axial images through the upper plane of the joint and the coracoid process. The humeral head is normally rounded at this level (Fig. 4.**52**). If prominent, the Hill–Sachs defect may be seen on the coronal images as well (Fig. 4.**53**).

An anterior dislocation which results in a tear of the glenoidal labrum is likely to damage the anterior capsule of the joint as well, unless

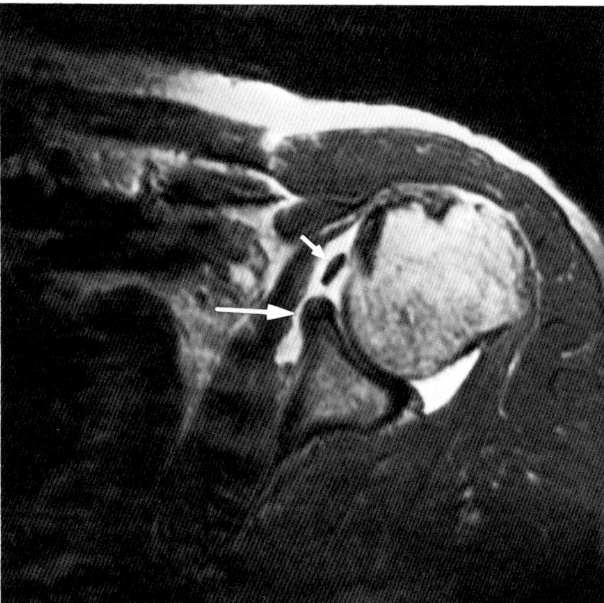

Fig. 4.**51** Axial T2 image (TR 2000/ TE 60). The anterior glenoidal labrum is hypertrophied (large arrow). A segment of the middle glenohumeral ligament is seen (small arrow)

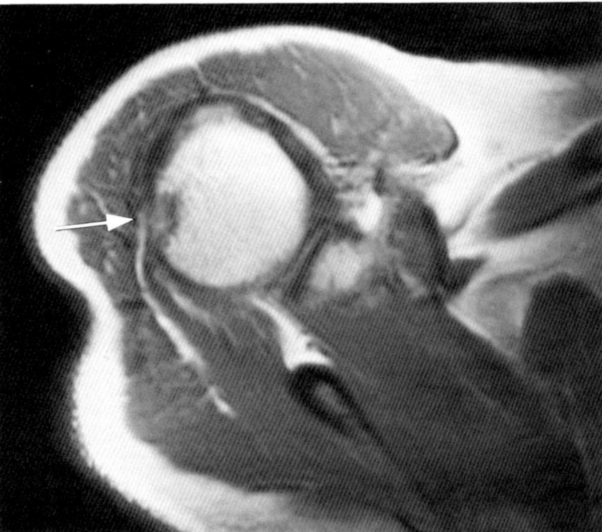

Fig. 4.**52** Axial proton-density image (TR 2000/TE 20). A Hill–Sachs defect is present on the posterolateral humeral head (arrow)

there is already a lax joint capsule or an unusually large opening between the joint and the subscapularis bursa (Rafii et al., 1986). It has been shown experimentally that with an anterior dislocation, the capsule tears most frequently in the elderly. In younger individuals, a separation of the capsule at its junction with the scapula is more likely to occur (Reeves, 1968). The capsule may tear a piece of attached labrum with it as it separates from the scapula. With concurrent tearing of the periosteum of the scapula and joint swelling, the capsule may heal with its attachment in a more medial position than originally, which will result in the medially capacious joint capsules of grades II and III. This condition can lead to a

Fig. 4.**53** Coronal proton-density image (TR 2000/TE 20). A Hill–Sachs defect is seen on the posterolateral humeral head (arrow)

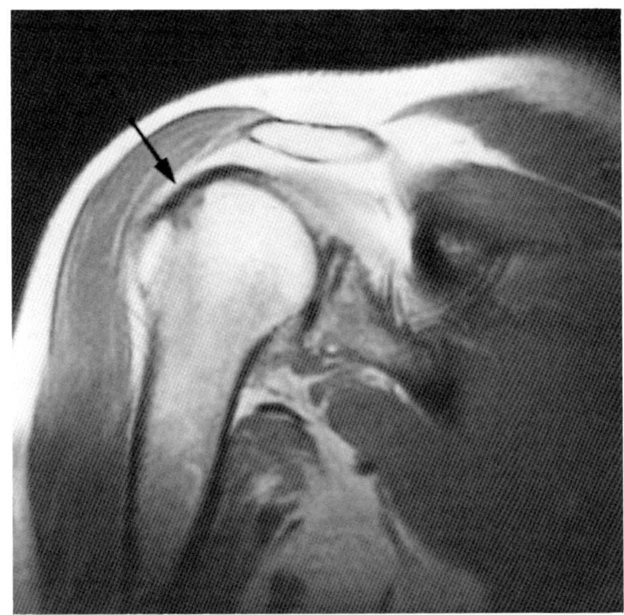

Fig. 4.**54** Axial T2 image (TR 2000/TE 60). Moderately medial attachment of the joint capsule to the scapula (arrow)

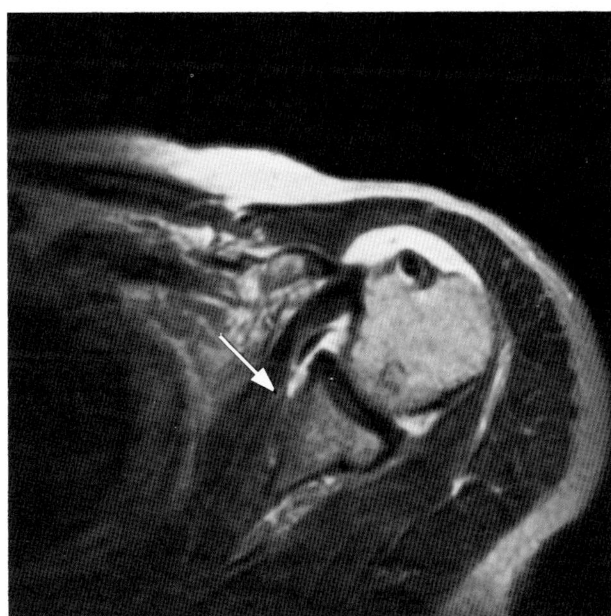

propensity for recurrent dislocation. Indeed, the joint capsule is presently considered more important for joint stability than the labrum (Rowe et al., 1978). This condition is best demonstrated on axial images (Figs. 4.**54**, 4.**55**). Differention of normal from abnormal is facilitated if an effusion distends the joint space (Figs. 4.**56**, 4.**57**). If little or no joint fluid is present, the capsule will be obscured by surrounding tissue and an abnormal medial attachment may be difficult recognize (see Fig. 4.**46b**). This is a potential disadvantage of MRI in comparison to computed tomographic (CT) arthrography. In the latter, air and contrast are injected into the joint space, which distends the joint, allowing identification of

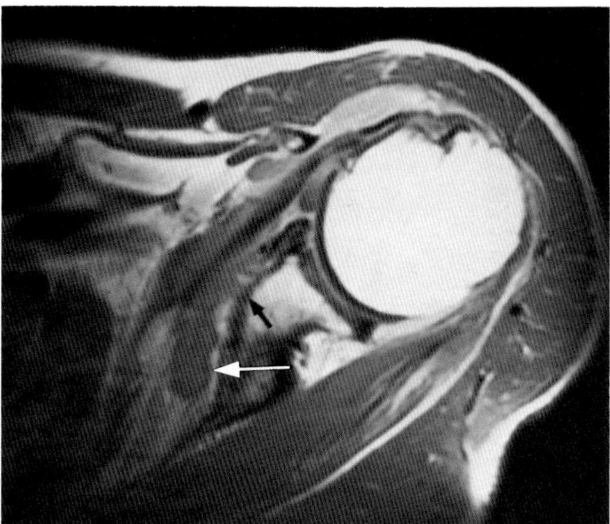

Fig. 4.**55a** Axial proton-density image (TR 2000/TE 20) and **b** axial T2 image (TR 2000/TE 60). There is a medially attaching joint capsule (small arrow in **a**). A medial extension of the joint under the subscapularis tendon increases the spaciousness of the anterior joint (large arrows in **a** and **b**)

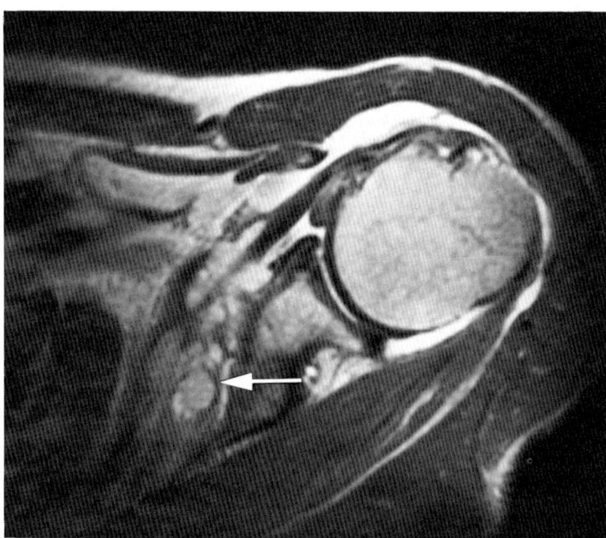

the site of anterior attachment (Fig. 4.**58**). Of course, this technique has the disadvantages of being an invasive procedure, using ionizing radiation, and allowing images of the shoulder only in the axial plane of the patient.

The subscapularis muscle extends across the shoulder joint anteriorly, and its tendon inserts on the lesser tuberosity. The muscle can be stretched and torn during an episode of dislocation. If a complete tear occurs, this will be seen best on axial views, with disruption of the muscle fibers adjacent to the anterior joint or detachment of the tendon from the humerus (Fig. 4.**59**). More frequently, only stretching or partial tearing will occur. If imaging is performed soon enough following the dislocation

Fig. 4.**56** Axial T2 image (TR 2000/TE 60). Medial attachment of the joint capsule is present, which is more easily seen because of the distention of the joint with fluid (arrow)

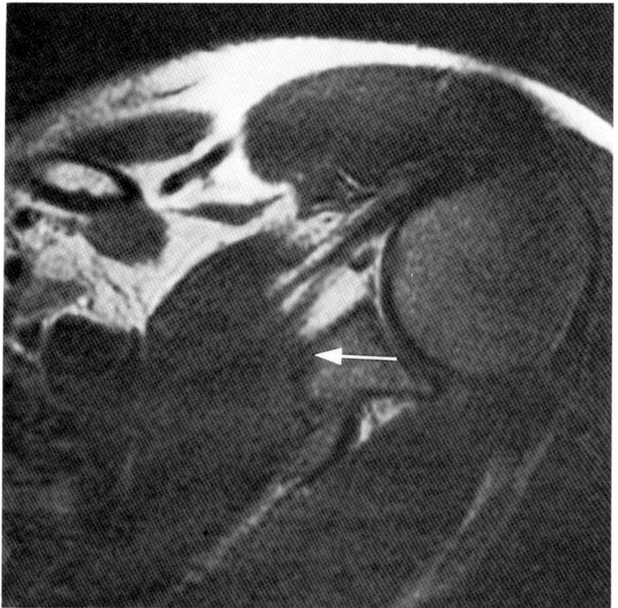

Fig. 4.**57** Axial T2 image (TR 2000/TE 60). In contrast to Fig. 4.**56**, this image depicts a joint also distended with fluid, but the capsule attaches in the normal position (arrow)

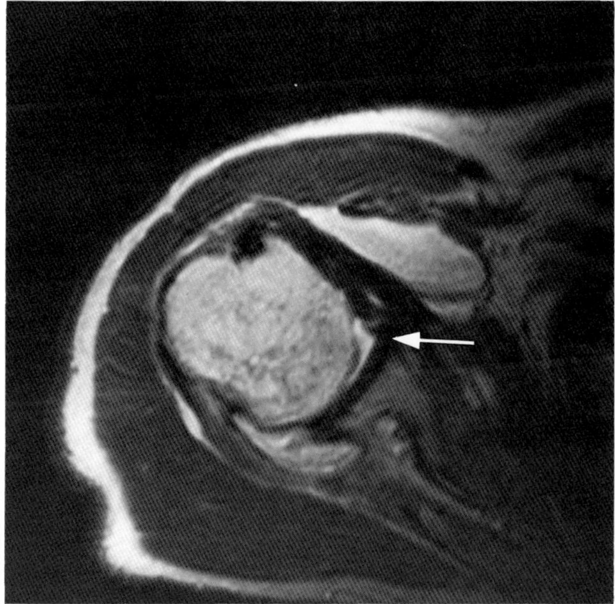

and reduction, edema with high signal on the T2 images may be evident in the muscle fibers or tendon. In more delayed examinations, the muscle fibers and/or tendon may appear lax and redundant. There may be fluid with distention in the subscapular bursa, which normally communicates with the joint space. The lateral muscle fibers may appear atrophic as well.

Injury involving any or all of the anterior shoulder structures may be seen following a single traumatic episode of dislocation. Once these injuries have occurred, the glenohumeral articulation is less well protected, and dislocation or subluxation may occur more easily. The joint capsule itself is now thought to be the most significant structure lending

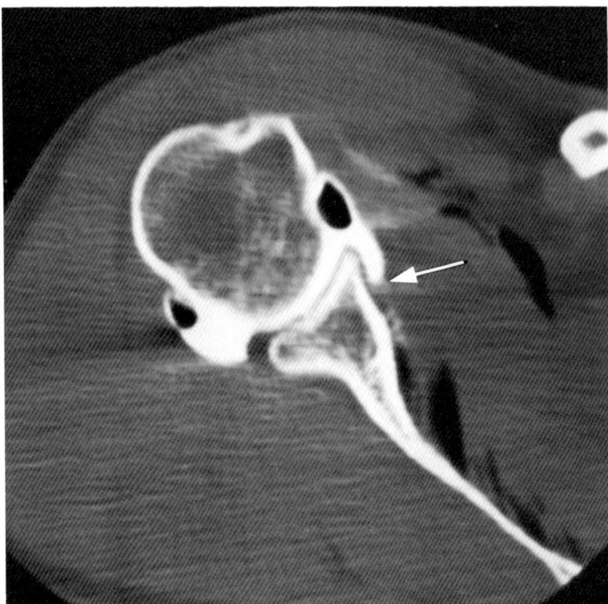

Fig. 4.**58** Axial view of a CT arthrogram of the shoulder. The injected air and contrast distend the joint space, allowing for identification of the type of anterior capsular attachment. This capsule attaches more medially than normal (arrow; Courtesy of Dr. Enrique Palacios, Macneal Hospital, Berwyn, Illinois)

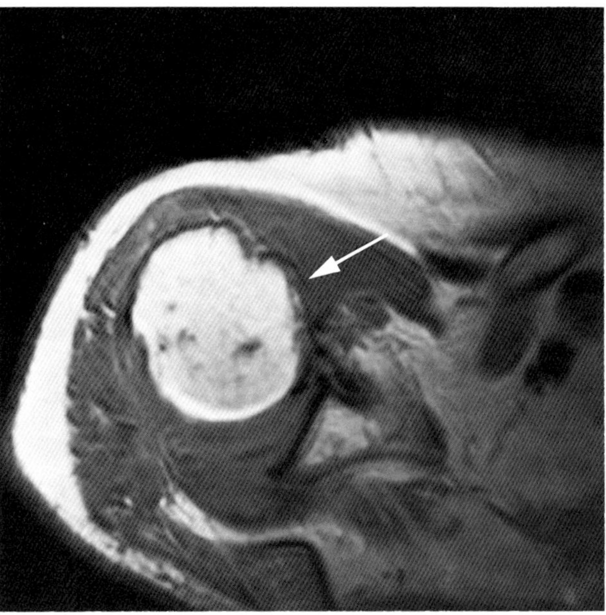

Fig. 4.**59** Axial proton-density image (TR 2000/TE 20). The subscapularis tendon was torn during an episode of anterior shoulder dislocation (arrow). The distal tendon attaching to the rim of the bicipital tendon groove is atrophic

shoulder stability; a glenoidal labrum or glenoid rim fracture plays a less important role in recurrent dislocation (Protzman, 1980; Rowe et al., 1978). The Hill–Sachs defect is also thought to be a factor in some cases (Rowe et al., 1978). A lax or deficient subscapularis muscle has been considered a factor (Symeonides, 1972; Fig. 4.**60**). In a series of 162 patients who had shoulder surgery within a 30-year period, Rowe and co-workers found a separation of the anterior capsule from the rim of the glenoid in 85 % of the cases, a tear of the glenoidal labrum with or without associated fracture of the glenoid rim in 73 %, and a Hill–Sachs deformity of the humeral head in 77 % (1978).

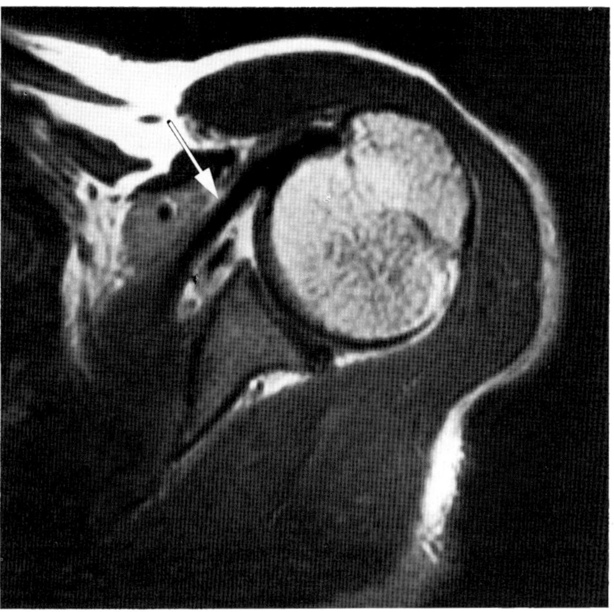

Fig. 4.**60** Axial T2 image (TR 2000/TE 60). A lax subscapularis tendon is present (arrow) with a capacious anterior joint space and the potential for anterior instability

Another type of unstable shoulder, but without a prior history of injury, is due to congenital laxity of the joint capsule and surrounding tendons. Patients with this condition may subluxate the shoulder at will and without pain. There is no evidence of prior trauma on the MR scan since there was no initiating dislocation to cause the condition. The MR scan shows no trauma-related abnormalities but may demonstrate redundancy of the joint capsule or subscapularis, particularly if there is sufficient joint fluid for distention. Early degenerative changes may be present. We have examined one patient, a 35-year-old woman with a subjective feeling of shoulder instability who was noted to have a small-diameter glenoid fossa (Fig. 4.**61**). Since no other abnormalities were observed, it was thought that the reduced contact between the humeral head and the glenoid was responsible for the presumed instability.

Posterior shoulder dislocations are much less frequent than anterior, constituting only about 4% of shoulder dislocations (Turek, 1984). The initiating trauma is a posterior force with the humeral head in internal rotation. There is a sudden sharp pain, but the arm is held in adduction and internal rotation. Conventional films can be difficult to interpret, as they may show only a subtle loss of the parallel alignment between the medial humeral head and the glenoid fossa. An oblique coronal view centered on the joint may reveal an overlap of the two structures and be diagnostic. A transaxillary view is usually impossible without general anesthesia since the patient cannot abduct the arm, without pain.

The injuries seen by MR after posterior dislocation correspond to those after anterior dislocation, but on the opposite side of the joint. The posterior labrum may be torn or the posterior rim of the glenoid fractured (Fig. 4.**62**). Since the joint capsule should always attach directly adjacent to the glenoid rim posteriorly, the observation of a more medial attachment is a good indication of posterior instability. Following a posterior dislocation, a

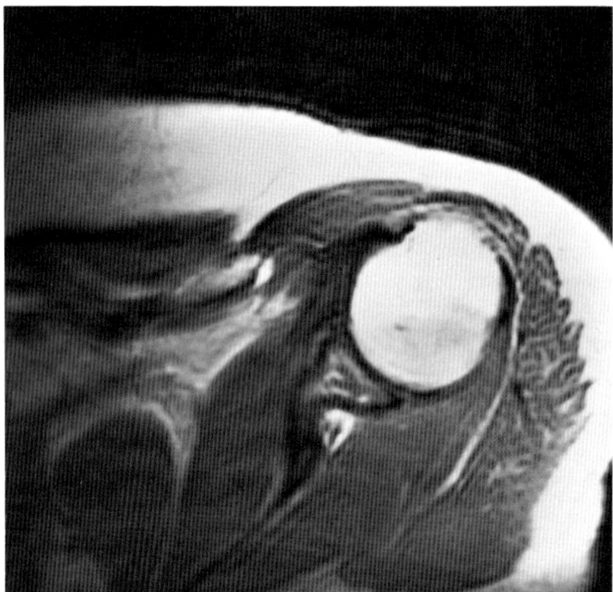

a

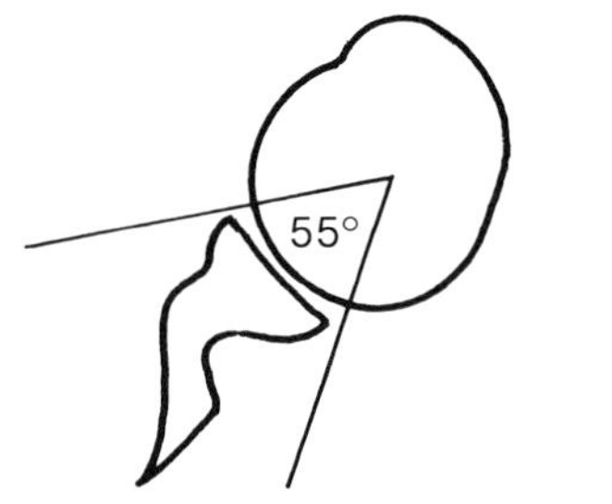

Fig. 4.**61a** Axial proton-density image (TR 2000/TE 20). The glenoid is smaller than normal in relation to the humeral head. It subtends an angle of 55° maximally of the circumference of the humeral head (**b**). An angle of 60° to 70° is normally observed

b

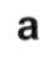

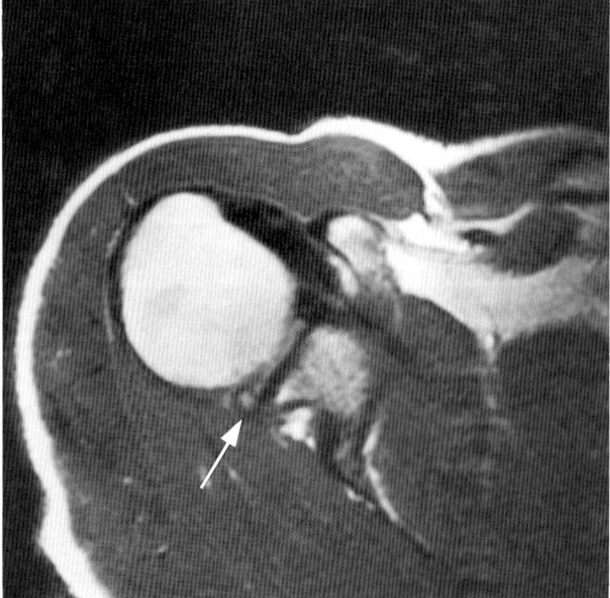

Fig. 4.**62** Axial T2 image (TR 2000/TE 60). The patient was a 30-year-old man with a history of previous posterior dislocation. He currently had extreme pain with internal rotation, particularly when putting his hand behind his back. The high signal due to a tear of the posterior glenoidal labrum is evident (arrow)

compression injury by the glenoid rim can result in a reverse Hill–Sachs defect seen on the anterior inferior aspect of the humeral head. With severe or recurrent dislocation, the infraspinatus may be torn or atrophic.

A tear of the inferior margin of the glenoidal labrum may result in recurrent inferior subluxation of the humeral head. This portion of the labrum is best seen in profile on the coronal sections.

MR imaging of the postoperative shoulder presents special interpretation problems because of the anatomical changes produced by surgery and the distortion of the MR signal in the presence of ferromagnetic surgical clips. The most frequent repair for shoulder impinge-

Fig. 4.**63**   Coronal proton-density image (TR 2000/TE 60). A tapered lateral aspect of the acromion process is seen after a previous acromioplasty to alleviate shoulder impingement syndrome (arrow)

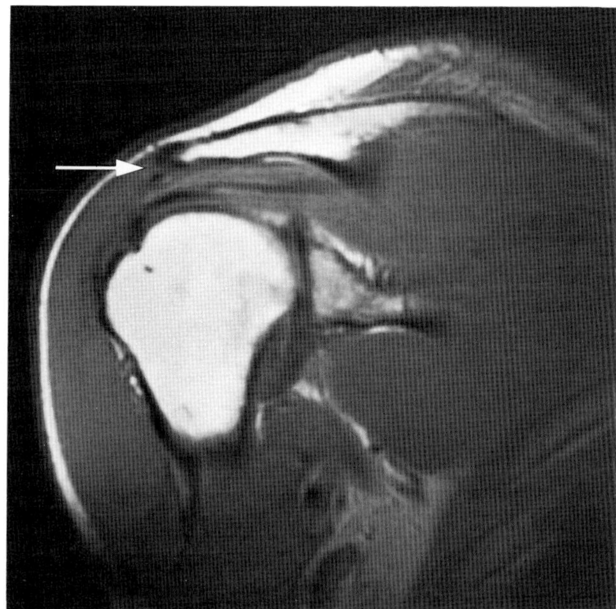

Fig. 4.**64**   Coronal T2 image (TR 2000/TE 60).There is a gap between the lateral clavicle and the acromion from a prior resection of the lateral clavicle to relieve shoulder impingement

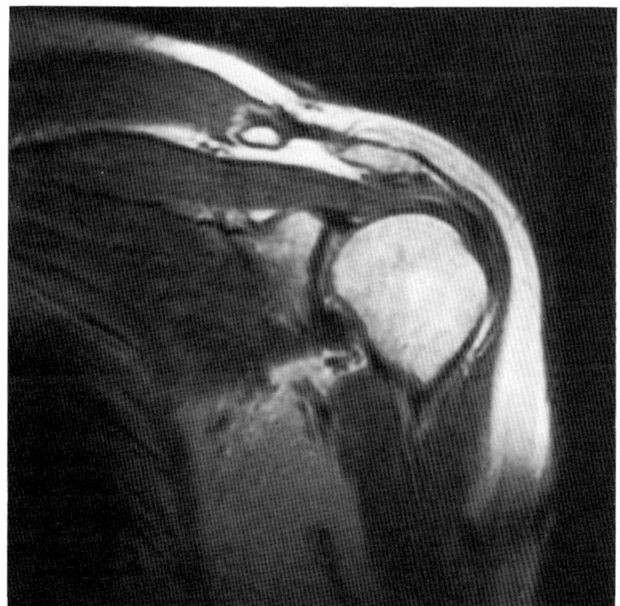

ment is an acromioplasty. This can be recognized by the smooth margin of the inferior acromion process anteriorly, with lateral tapering of the acromion (Fig. 4.**63**). There is a wide space between the humeral head and the acromion. If the acromioclavicular joint was the site of impingement, a partial osteotomy around the joint may been seen (Fig. 4.**64**).

After repair of a torn supraspinatus tendon, small low-signal dots representing suture material may be seen. Reoccurrence of pain following surgery can be due to avascular necrosis of the humeral head (Fig. 4.**65**). Recurrent anterior shoulder instability may be surgically corrected by an anterior capsulorrhaphy (Fig. 4.**66**).

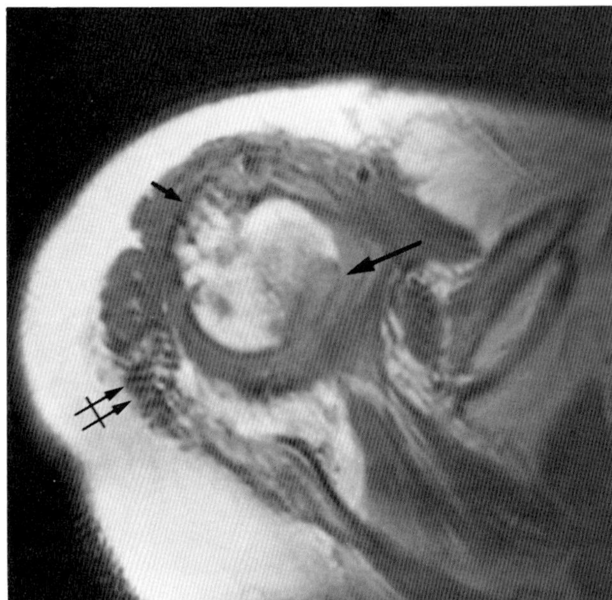

a

Fig. 4.**65a** Axial proton-density image (TR 2000/TE 20). Small low-signal dots are due to suture material of a surgical repair for a complete tear of the supraspinatus tendon (small arrow). There are also sutures in the deltoid muscle (double arrow). There is avascular necrosis of the medial side of the humeral head (large arrow). This is intermediate signal intensity, in contrast to the normal high signal from fatty bone marrow

b Coronal T2 image (TR 2000/TE 60). The thin surgically repaired supraspinatus tendon is seen (small arrow). The avascular necrosis of the humeral head has a high signal intensity on the T2 image (large arrow)

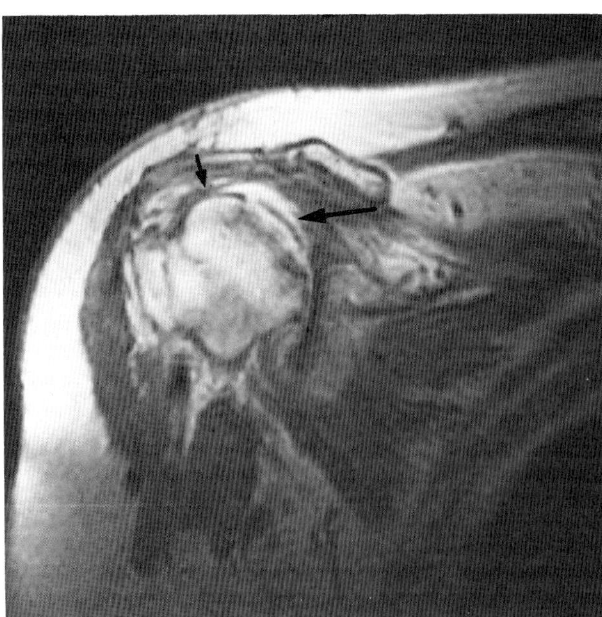

b

Fig. 4.**66** Axial proton-density image (TR 2000/TE 20). There has been an anterior capsulorrhaphy. The joint capsule is thickened anteriorly, and low-signal dots due to suture material are present

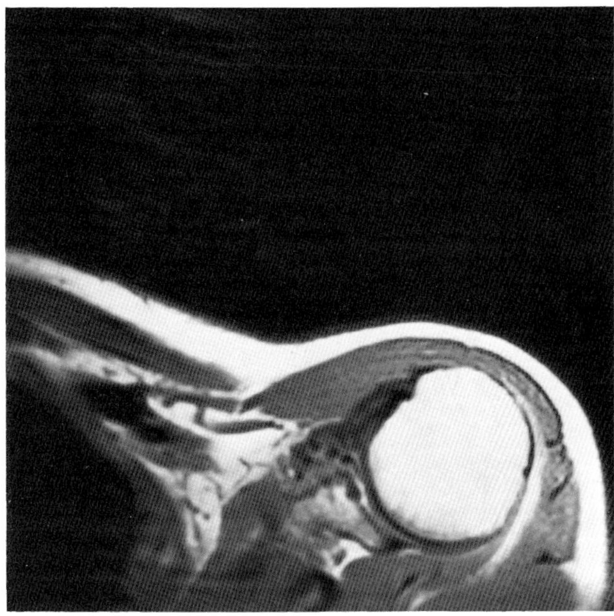

References

Bankart ASB. The pathology and treatment of recurrent dislocation of the shoulder. Br J Surg 1938; 26:23-9.

Burk DL, Karasick D, Kurtz AB, et al. Rotator cuff tears: Prospective comparison of MR imaging with arthrography, sonography and surgery. Am J Roentgenol 1989; 153:87–92.

DePalma AF. Surgery of the shoulder. 3rd ed. Philadelphia: Lippincott, 1983:55–60, 512–58.

Kieft G, Bloem J, Rozing P, Obermann W. MR imaging of recurrent anterior dislocation of the shoulder: comparison with CT arthrography. Am J Roentgenol 1988:150:1083–7.

Moseley HF, Overgaard B. The anterior capsular mechanism in recurrent anterior dislocation of the shoulder: morphological and clinical studies with special reference to the glenoid labrum and glenohumeral ligaments. J Bone Joint Surg (Br) 1962;44:913–27.

Neer C. Anterior acromioplasty for the chronic impingement syndrome in the shoulder. J Bone Joint Surg (Am) 1972;54:41–50.

Neer C. Impingement lesions. Clin Orthop 1983;173:70–7.

Neer C, Welsh RP. The shoulder in sports. Orthop Clin North Am 1977;8:583–91.

Post M. Physical examination of the shoulder. In: Physical examination of the musculoskeletal system. Chicago, London: Yearbook, 1987:13–55.

Protzman R. Anterior instability of the shoulder. J Bone Joint Surg (Am) 1980;62:909–18.

Rafii M, Firooznia H, Golimbu C, Minkoff J, Bonamo J. CT arthrography of capsular structures of the shoulder. Am J Roentgenol 1986;146:361–7.

Reeves B. Experiments of the tensile strength of the anterior capsular structures of the shoulder in man. J Bone Joint Surg (Br) 1968;50:858–65.

Rothman RH, Marvel JP Jr, Heppenstall RB. Anatomic considerations in the glenohumeral joint. Orthop Clin North Am 1975;6:341–52.

Rowe C, Patel D, Southmayd W. The Bankart procedure. J Bone Joint Surg (Am) 1978;60:1–16.

Salter R. Fractures and joint injuries in adults and musculoskeletal disorders. In: Textbook of disorders and injuries of the musculoskeletal system. 2nd ed. Baltimore, London: Williams & Wilkins, 1983:501–5,240–5.

Seeger LL, Gold RH, Bassett LW. Shoulder instability: evaluation with MR imaging. Radiology 1988;168:695–7.

Seeger LL, Gold RH, Bassett LW, Ellman H. Shoulder impingement syndrome: MR findings in 53 shoulders. Am J Roentgenol 1988;150:343–7.

Symeonides P. The significance of the subscapularis muscle in the pathogenesis of recurrent anterior dislocation of the shoulder. J Bone Joint Surg (Br) 1972;54:476–83.

Townley CO. The capsular mechanism in recurrent dislocation of the shoulder. J Bone Joint Surg (Am) 1950;32:370–80.

Turek S. The shoulder. In: Orthopaedics: principles and their applications. 4th ed. Philadelphia: Lippincott, 1984:920–66.

Turkel SJ, Panio MW, Marshall JL. Stabilizing mechanisms preventing anterior dislocation of the glenohumeral joint. J Bone Joint Surg (Am) 1981;63:1208–17.

Zlatkin M, Reicher M, Kellerhouse L, et al. The painful shoulder: MR imaging of the glenohumeral joint. J Comput Assist Tomogr 1988;12:995–1001.

Zlatkin M, Dalinka M, Kressel H. Magnetic resonance imaging of the shoulder. Magn Reson Q 1989;5:3–22.

Zohn DA. Crossmatching clinical diagnoses with treatment principles. In: Musculoskeletal pain: diagnosis and treatment. 2nd ed. Boston, Toronto: Little, Brown, 1988:165–79.

5 Case Studies

The following case studies are of patients who presented to me with complaints of shoulder pain. They represent some of the most common types of shoulder pathology that the clinician may encounter.

The photographs were obtained during arthroscopy. In them, the glenoid articular surface is oriented horizontally, as the patients are in the lateral decubitus position during surgery.

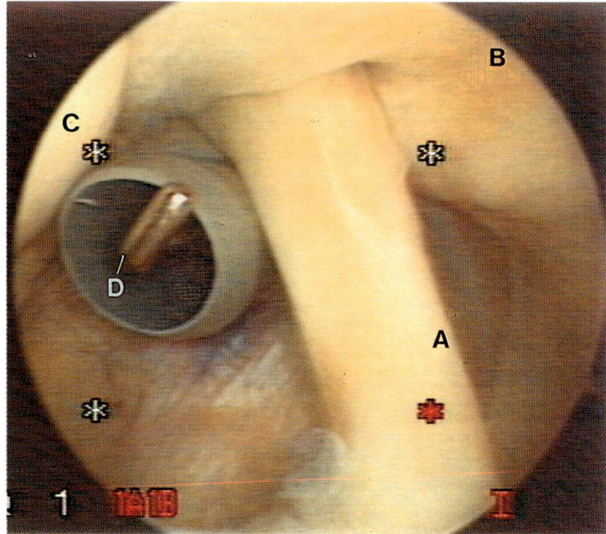

Fig. 5.1   A normal biceps tendon (A) and undersurface of the rotator cuff (B). The humeral head is to the left (C). A plastic cannula and metal probe utilized in this procedure are also visualized (D)

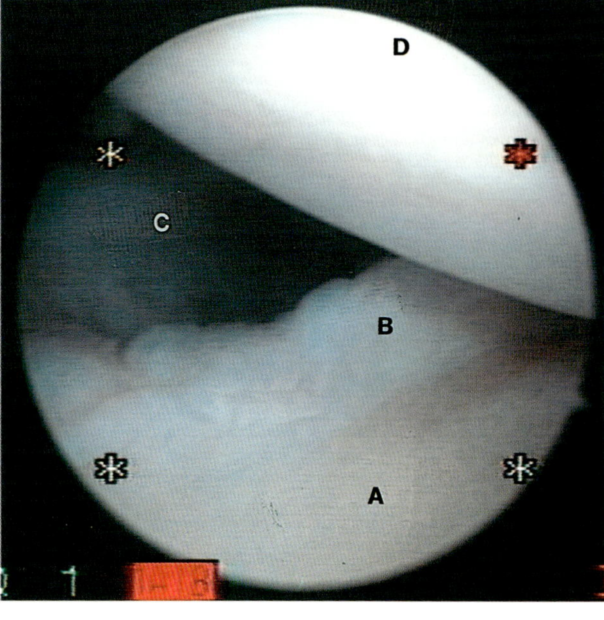

Fig. 5.2   This demonstrates a normal anterior glenoid ligament (A) and anterior labrum—inferior glenohumeral ligament complex (B). The middle glenohumeral ligament lies anteriorly (C). The humeral head is to the right (D)

Normal anatomy is shown in Figures 5.**1–4**.

Fig. 5.**3** This demonstrates the middle glenohumeral ligament (A). Note that it is anterior to the inferior glenohumeral ligament–labrum complex (B) and inserts medially on the glenoid neck. The subscapularis is also visualized (C). The humeral head is to the right (D)

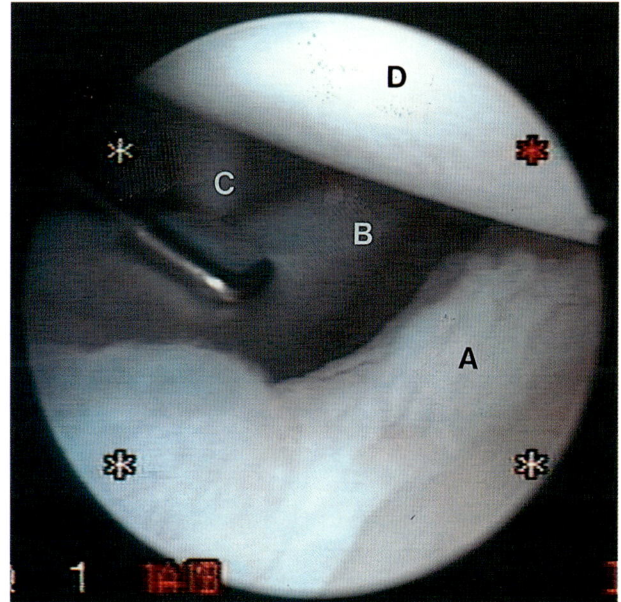

Fig. 5.**4** The normal "bare" area on the posterior surface of the humeral head (A) should not be confused with a Hill–Sachs defect, an indentation fracture seen with anterior instability. The rotator cuff and its insertion is superior (B) and the remainder of the articular surface is seen inferiorly here (C)

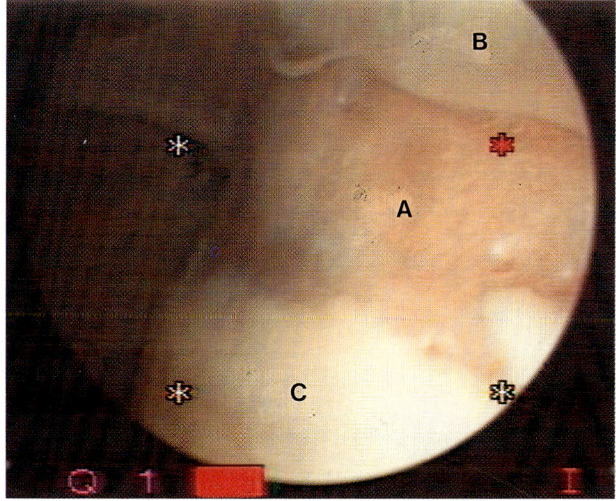

Case 1. This patient is a racquetball instructor who presented with complaints of shoulder pain with overhead activities. He had maximal tenderness at the anterior edge of the acromion. Pain was noted with resistive testing of the rotator cuff in abduction with maximal internal rotation of the arm (Figs. 3.**1**, 3.**2**). His MR image showed subacromial impingement and a partial rotator cuff tear. Arthroscopy was performed after failure with conservative treatment including nonsteroidal anti-inflammatory medication, subacromial anti-inflammatory injection, and physical therapy (Fig. 5.**5a**).

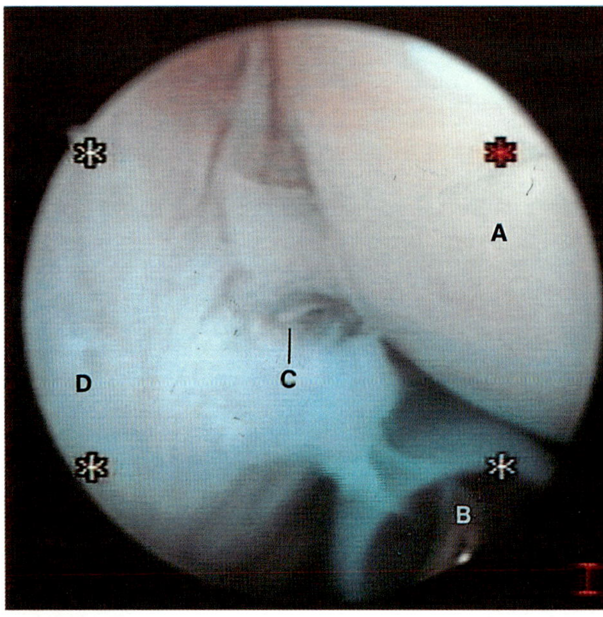

Fig. 5.**5a**   The humeral head is to the right here (A) and the cannula and metal probe used in the procedure are located inferiorly (B). A small partial-thickness tear is noted on the articular surface of the superior rotator cuff tendon (C). Normal tendon is also seen (D; for a comparable MR image, see Fig. 4.**16**)

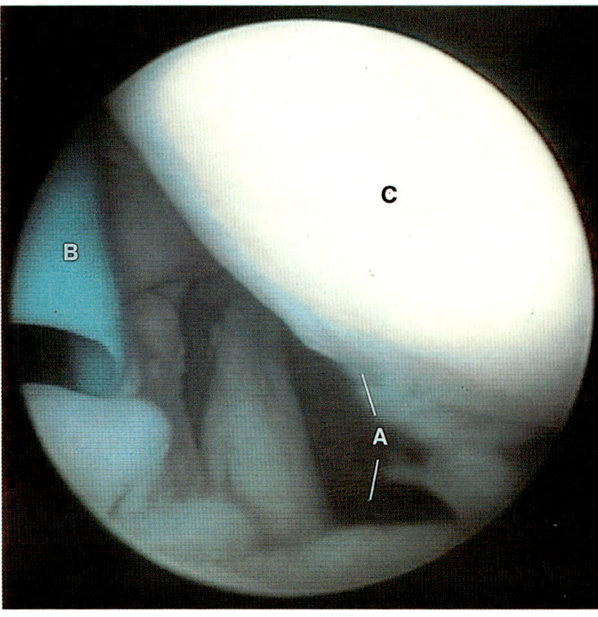

Fig. 5.**5b**   This is another patient with an MR image that showed a complete but small tear with normal surrounding rotator cuff tendon. Arthroscopy showed a small complete tear (A). The subacromial space is seen through the defect. The normal biceps tendon is retracted by the inflow cannula and is partially visualized (B). The humeral head is to the right (C; for a comparable MR image, see Fig. 4.**21**)

Case 2. This is an older patient. He is a fireman who complained of severe pain with arm elevation. He demonstrated significant weakness with both resisted abduction in internal rotation and with resisted external rotation.

He did not respond to conservative treatment. An MR image showed a complete rotator cuff tear with retraction of the tendon. Attempts to repair the tendon were unsuccessful due to the large size of this tear (Fig. 5.**6a**).

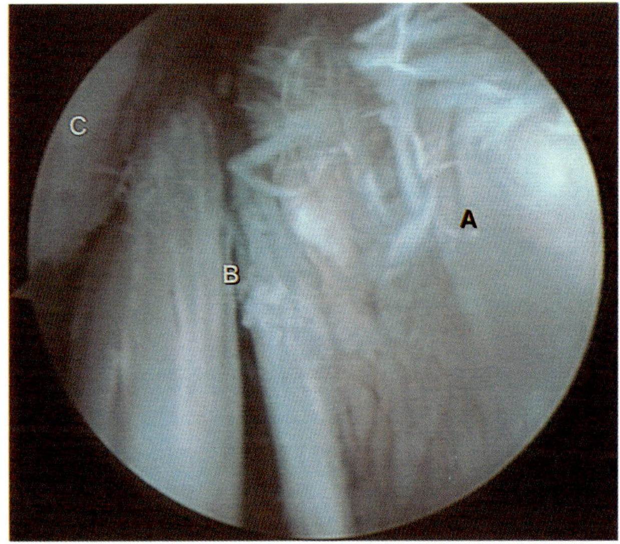

Fig. 5.**6a** The frayed undersurface of the acromion is visualized from inside the glenohumeral joint (A). Since there is no rotator cuff tendon tissue present, there is free communication between the glenohumeral joint and the subacromial space. The intra-articular portion of the biceps tendon is frayed and split longitudinally (B), and is noted adjacent to the humeral head (C; cf. Fig. 5.**1**)

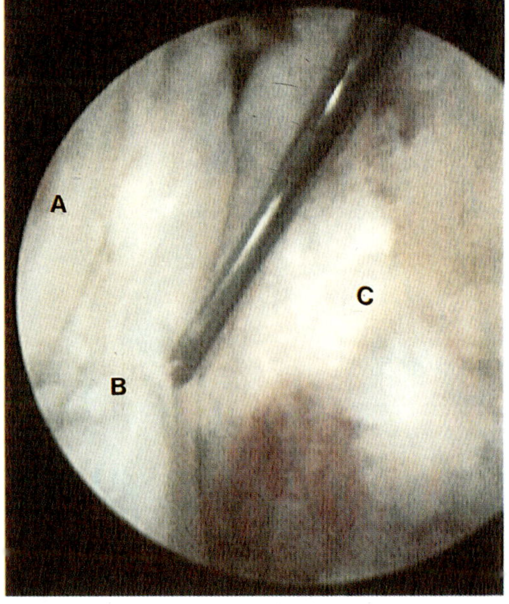

Fig. 5.**6b** This is another patient with a large complete tear. The humeral head is to the left (A) and the needle is on the retracted end of the tendon (B). The undersurface of the acromion is frayed and worn (C; for a comparable MR image, see Fig. 4.**24**)

Case 3. This is a collegiate baseball pitcher who noted progressive pain in his throwing shoulder. He had a positive apprehension test (Figs. 3.**4**, 3.**5**), and pain with resisted abduction and external rotation. An MR image showed a torn anterior labrum (Fig. 5.**7**).

Case 4. This recreational athlete also had a history of instability. He did not respond to conservative treatment and his MR image showed a Bankart defect with a fracture of the anterior glenoid (Figs. 5.**8**, 5.**9**).

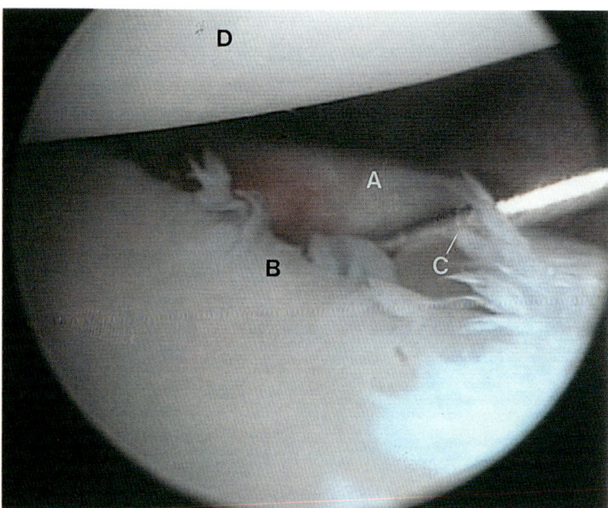

Fig. 5.**7**   The Bankart lesion, a detached anterior labrum–inferior glenohumeral ligament complex is noted here (A). The glenoid demonstrates minor fraying anteriorly (B). A metal probe is in the defect (C). The humeral head lies superiorly and has a normal appearance (D). This patient also had a partial-thickness tear on the articular surface of the rotator cuff (cf. Fig. 5.**2**)

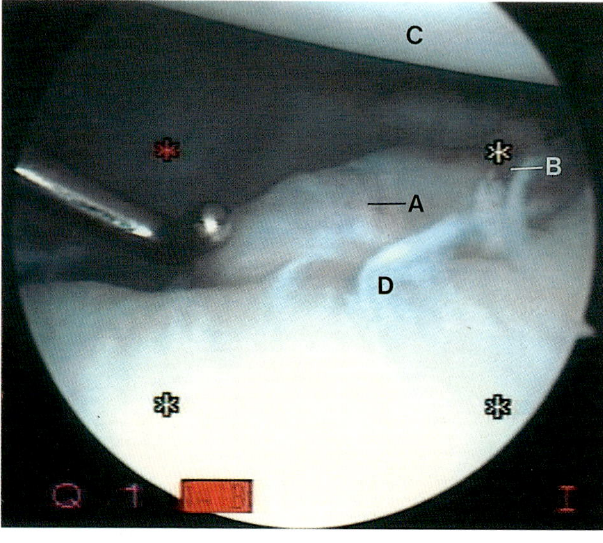

Fig. 5.**8**   A fracture of the anterior rim of the glenoid (A). The inferior glenohumeral ligament remained attached to the fragment and displaced with it medially on the glenoid neck (B). The humeral head appears normal anteriorly (C) and the glenoid shows some minor fraying anteriorly (D; for a comparable MR image, see Fig. 4.**50**)

Case 5. This patient is a wrestler from Hungary who had won an Olympic gold medal. He dislocated his shoulder 4 years later while attempting to win another medal. He could not resume his sport following conservative treatment due to his disability. MRI demonstrated a detached anterior glenoidal labrum (Fig. 5.**10**).

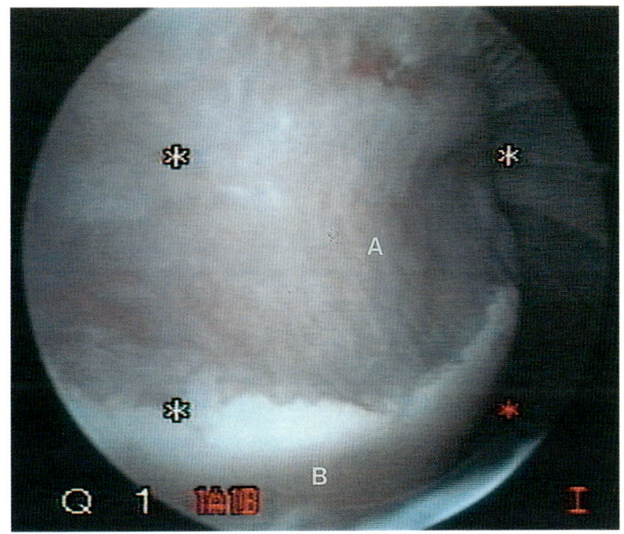

Fig. 5.**9**   This same patient showed evidence of anterior instability when his humeral head was visualized completely. A large indentation fracture (Hill–Sachs lesion) is noted (A; cf. Fig. 5.**4**). Normal articular cartilage is noted below (B). This patient had an open repair to stabilize his shoulder (for a comparable MR image, see Fig. 4.**52**)

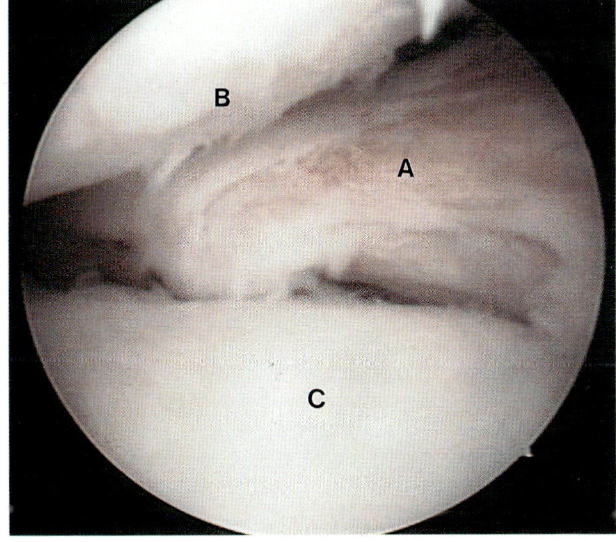

Fig. 5.**10**   A large Bankart lesion is noted with detachment of the entire anterior labrum (A). The humeral head shows some fraying (B). The glenoid surface is normal (C). This patient had an arthroscopic labrum repair with intra-articular suturing. He recently won the European Championship

Case 6. This patient trades at the Board of Exchange. He had pain and a catching sensation in his dominant shoulder when he worked. MRI showed multiple lesions in the glenohumeral joint which appeared to be cartilaginous in nature (Fig. 5.**11**).

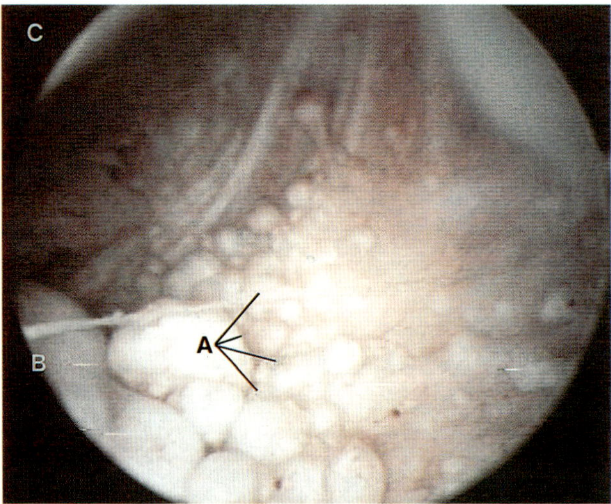

Fig. 5.**11a** Arthroscopy revealed synovial chondromatosis with multiple loose bodies and abnormal synovium throughout the shoulder. Here in the inferior recess of the glenohumeral joint, pedular lesions and loose bodies are noted (A). The glenoid is to the left (B) and the humeral head is just barely seen (C)

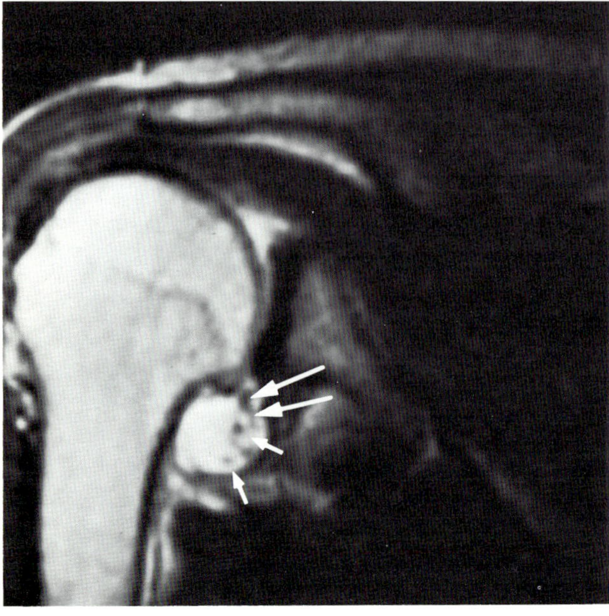

Fig. 5.**11b** MRI of the same patient demonstrates the synovial chondromas as multiple round, low-signal dots (arrows) against the high-signal background of joint effusion

6 Treatment of Shoulder Disorders

Shoulder disorders, like many other musculo-skeletal injuries, should be initially treated conservatively. This may include the use of heat or cold, nonsteroidal anti-inflammatory medications, as well as some rest. Complete restriction of activities, however, is rarely necessary.

Physical therapy is helpful in advanced cases which do not respond to simple treatment. The therapist has many treatment modalities at his or her disposal which are designed to help alleviate pain and aid the repair process.

Relief of pain should be the primary goal of the treating physician. Nonsteroidal medications are helpful since they reduce pain by decreasing the inflammation that causes discomfort. This may facilitate early mobilization of the shoulder and may help avoid posttraumatic loss of motion.

Mobilization of the shoulder is helpful and should be performed with patients with instability who may have developed capsular tightness as a result of long-standing instability. Mobilization may also be helpful to patients with impingement of the rotator cuff by the acromion.

Range of motion exercises should be performed as soon as possible after injury due to the propensity of the shoulder to lose motion following trauma. This includes pendulum exercises initially and later, passive range of motion exercises. Active range of motion exercises are performed later, when the patient is able to tolerate increased motion. Strengthening exercises are difficult for the patient initially, although isometric exercises are often possible. With time, strengthening within the full range of active motion should be possible. Shoulder strengthening exercises should initially involve the internal and external rotators (Fig. 6.1). These are comfortably performed at the side and are particularly important in patients with impingement, since the rotator cuff, which functions in internal and external rotation, is also an important humeral head

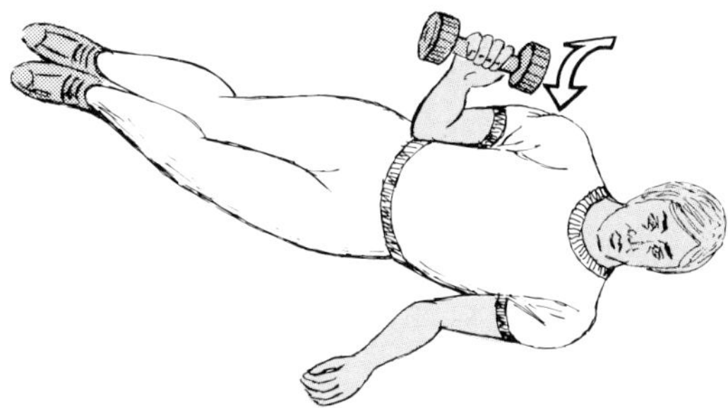

Fig. 6.1 Strengthening the external rotators is best performed with the patient on his or her side

depressor. Strengthening this muscle will therefore decrease subacromial impingement (Fig. 6.2). Patients who, in an attempt to regain abduction, strengthen the deltoid excessively at the expense of the rotator cuff musculature will develop increased impingement due to the proximal migration of the humeral head produced by the deltoid.

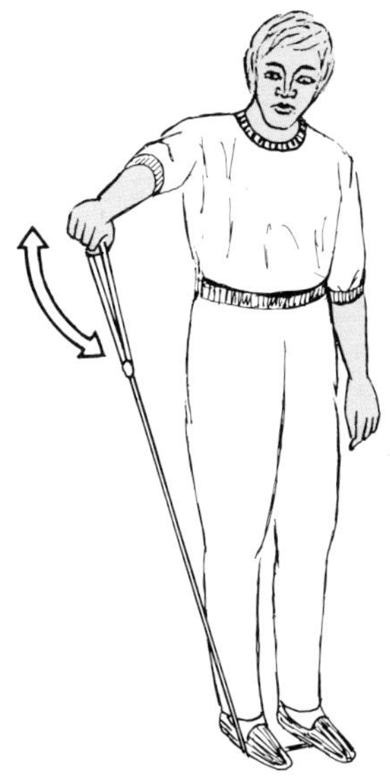

Fig. 6.2 Strengthening of the rotator cuff by abducting the shoulder in internal rotation. Elastic devices or light weights (less than 2.25 kg) are used

The scapular musculature should also be strengthened, since weakness and elongation of these muscles allow downward rotation of the scapula and increased impingement by the acromion.

Strengthening the internal and external rotators is important within instability. Current emphasis on the association between anterior instability and impingement has increased our appreciation of the fact that rotator cuff strengthening is an important component of the rehabilitation of anterior instability.

Posterior and multidirectional instabilities are less common than anterior or anteroinferior shoulder instabilities. These patients should be treated with a strengthening program. This is particularly important in patients who can voluntarily dislocate their shoulders posteriorly or patients with generalized soft tissue laxity.

Conservative treatment is successful in many patients with shoulder injuries. This should be attempted prior to proceeding with surgery. Patients for whom conservative treatment does not suceed and who therefore require surgery benefit from preoperative conditioning since it expedites the postoperative recovery.

Some patients, however, are not candidates for conservative treatment. Fractures, particularly open fractures, should be treated surgically. Anterior dislocations, particularly in young patients, may not respond to conservative treatment and have been shown to have a high recurrence rate.

Impingement and recurrent instability which does not respond to conservative treatment may require surgery. Arthroscopic surgery is helpful in these patients since it allows visualization of the intra-articular and bursal pathology. It also permits treatment of lesions noted during the procedure. Rotator cuff tears due to impingement may be seen on the bursal surface of the rotator cuff tendon. Anterior instability causes a tensile failure of the rotator cuff. These tears are seen on the articular surface of its tendon.

Partial or complete but small (less than 1 cm) rotator cuff tears, particularly in older patients, may be treated with arthroscopic debridement and subacromial decompression. This procedure includes acromioplasty and coracoacromial ligament release. Arthroscopic treatment may also be helpful in patients with massive rotator cuff tears, since the results of aggressive treatment of these patients has been variable.

Large tears (greater than 1 cm) or smaller tears in younger athletes require repair. This may be performed arthroscopically with new instrumentation available now, but long-term results of these techniques are not yet available. Most orthopedic surgeons are familiar with conventional open repairs of these tears which require mobilization and advancement of the rotator cuff. Repairs which are so tenuous that they require splinting in abduction will most likely not be successful. Some failures of rotator cuff repairs are due to degenerative arthritis of the acromioclavicular joint which may not have been appreciated initially. Distal clavicle resection may be required in these patients.

Arthroscopic evaluation prior to open repair in patients with large rotator cuff tears is useful for debriding intra-articular lesions which cannot be seen during the open procedure and may compromise the postoperative result. Arthroscopy also allows evaluation of the extent of the intra-articular degenerative arthritis.

The operative treatment of instability has also undergone a rapid transformation in the past few years. The standard procedures for recurrent instability are those which require arthrotomy with capsular tightening. Some procedures involve shortening internal or external rotators, which result in postoperative loss of motion. This decrease in motion may be acceptable to some patients, but may excessively limit motion in athletes participating in sports requiring overhead throwing. Other procedures involve transferring muscles and the use of screws or staples, which may loosen and migrate. Newer methods utilize fixation materials with attached sutures which are wholly contained within the bone. This prevents migration of the implant.

Arthroscopic procedures for instability have evolved in an attempt to correct the instability without causing postoperative loss of motion.

Arthroscopic stapling of a detached capsule has been performed in some patients with instability (Gross, 1989). Loosening of the staple and intra-articular migration can lead to destruction of the articular surfaces.

Intra-articular suturing techniques are attractive since they do not require metallic fixation material. They may, however, require drilling tunnels through the glenoid neck and into the infraspinous fossa. This may injure the suprascapular nerve. Newer methods utilize absorbable fixation materials which can be used to reattach a torn capsule to the glenoid.

Arthroscopic stabilization procedures are attractive and result in less postoperative loss of motion. The failure rate from these types of procedures, however, has been high in the contact athlete. With modifications of present methods, they may become the treatment of choice in this group of patients.

In conclusion, the treatment of most shoulder disorders should, if possible, be conservative. Operative treatment may be needed in some patients but it is associated within creased morbidity (Norwood and Fowler, 1989). Although arthroscopic procedures have less morbidity than conventional shoulder surgery, purely diagnostic arthroscopy should nevertheless be performed only on a limited basis. Noninvasive procedures, such as MRI, should be used to diagnose shoulder disorders and assist with preoperative planning (Gross et al., 1990). Imaging techniques are very helpful, but they should not be used as a substitute for a careful history and physical examination.

References

Gross ML et al. Magnetic resonance imaging of the glenoid labrum. Am J Sportsmed 1990;18(3):229–34.
Gross RM. Arthroscopic staple capsulorrhaphy: does it work? Am J Sportsmed 1989;17(4):495–500.
Norwood LA, Fowler HL. Rotator cuff tears: a shoulder arthroscopy complication. Am J Sportsmed 1989; 17(6):837–41.

Index

A